Praise for *The Raw Food Detox Diet*

"An easy, ultra-effective diet you're gonna love!"

—*Woman's World*

"In clear, inspiring language, Rose explains how your body responds to various foods and food combinations. This book helps you put the science of enzymes to work for better health."

—*Total Health*

"The true 'anti-fad' diet . . . There's no deprivation with this regimen—just satisfaction, with slimming results."

—*Hamptons Magazine*

"Another great diet alternative, particularly for those who prefer a more holistic, food-based approach to weight loss."

—*eDiets.com*

ERGY ★ RAW FOOD LIFE FORCE ENERGY ★ RAW

ALSO BY NATALIA ROSE

The Raw Food Detox Diet

★ RAW FOOD LIFE FORCE ENERGY ★

ENTER A TOTALLY NEW STRATOSPHERE OF WEIGHT LOSS, BEAUTY, AND HEALTH

Natalia Rose

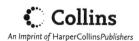

Collins

An Imprint of HarperCollinsPublishers

For my Father and his eternal music.

For the resplendent future of all humankind.

A hardcover edition of this book was published in 2007 by HarperCollins Publishers.

HarperCollins books may be purchased for educational, business, or sales promotional use. For information please write: Special Markets Department, HarperCollins Publishers, 10 East 53rd Street, New York, NY 10022.

First Collins paperback edition published 2008

Designed by Kris Tobiassen

The Library of Congress has catalogued the hardcover edition as follows:

Rose, Natalia.
     Raw food life force energy : enter a whole new stratosphere of weight loss, beauty, and health / Natalia Rose.—1st ed.
        p. cm.
     ISBN-13: 978-0-06-117618-0
     1. Raw food diet.   2. Reducing diets.   3. Health.   I. Title.

RM237.5.R68 2007

ISBN 978-0-06-134465-7 (pbk.)   2006051006

08 09 10 11 12 RRD 10 9 8 7 6 5 4 3 2 1

ACKNOWLEDGMENTS

My heart wells up with gratitude when I look back on all the support I have received through the process of developing this book.

Thank you to my clients and readers—you are a constant source of inspiration. Your spirited way of embracing the ideas and applications behind my practice and your daily success stories drive me to do all I can to get this message out to as many people as possible. Many thanks for your part in spreading the word!

I could never have done this if it hadn't been for one particularly important person, Angela Arias, who has cared for my children for many years, enabling me to continue my practice and write knowing they were always safe and surrounded by love. I extend my deepest gratitude to her for this gift of peace of mind.

Thandi and Tommy, thank you so much for your patience. You two are the greatest!

Lawrence, you are the only home I will ever need. Thank you for being "the last good husband" and the greatest father to our children.

This book would never have been possible if not for the brilliance of forward-thinking quantum physicists and electromagnetic field researchers. Richard Gerber and Valerie Hunt, your research was particularly inspiring to me. Thank you for living your life purposes so we all could benefit from your knowledge!

A great big thank you to Bruce Tainio for contributing so much of his time and reviewing my earliest draft. He gave me time and attention that he didn't even have time to give. Bruce, I want you to know how deeply grateful I am to you for sharing your knowledge about vibrations, electromagnetics, and the future of agriculture. Finding you was an incredible gift and the answer to a long search for answers. You are a genius.

Nicola Robins, you have provided indescribable support for my growth over the years. My life and vision are so much richer because of you.

I want to acknowledge a source of guidance that has come to me from the realm of spirit. There are many ideas and epiphanies that came to me seemingly from out of the blue. But I know they were divinely sent. I am deeply humbled and enriched by this benevolent presence that gifts me with a constant flow of information and inspiration.

Many thanks to Ibrahim Bengay of The Raw Bakery and Sarma Melngailis of Pure Food and Wine restaurant for sharing their delicious recipes in this book. They are two of the brightest stars in raw food, and I am grateful that they took the time to offer their recipes and support.

Gil Jacobs, you are my teacher who has been with me every step of the way. You are a part of the healing that will take place in every single person affected by this book. You are such a humble teacher, yet you have inspired and helped heal more people than you will ever know. You are a gift to us all!

Mark Sayers and Christy Ferer, I will always remember all you have done for me.

A very special thank you to Gerardo Somoza and Richard Ljoenes for bringing all their artistic vitality to the cover design. Anna Bliss, editor extraordinaire: you are the one behind the scenes who made this whole project unfold as it was destined to. In addition to your incredible focus, innate talent, and impeccable instincts, you are a joy to be around and have made the process of this, our second book together, an absolute pleasure.

Judith Regan: you can't possibly know what an inspiration you are to me. In your world, the biggest dreams—and only the biggest dreams—become reality. I absolutely love you!

"Vibrational Medicine is Einsteinian Medicine, since it is Einstein's equation which gives us the key insight toward understanding that energy and matter are one and the same thing."

—RICHARD GERBER,
VIBRATIONAL MEDICINE

CONTENTS

PART III: RAW FOOD LIFE FORCE ENERGY RECIPES

FOREWORD

VIKTORAS KULVINSKAS

In my forty years within the natural health movement, I've been blessed to witness the living food lifestyle spread its wings and soar. When I started the Hippocrates Health Institute with Dr. Ann Wigmore in the 1960s, "raw" and "living" were not words commonly associated with the way we eat. I developed a living foods program, a radically new paradigm at the time, which demonstrated unquestionable healing powers. One by one people would arrive at the Institute with grave illnesses and depart revitalized by the simple preparations created from the uncooked bounty of nature.

Since that time, while numerous health fads have come and gone, the healing power of natural, raw food, and its enzymatic powers have withstood the test of time. While for many people physical healing is satisfying enough, I have always dreamed that the raw food lifestyle would also help people realize that they are all deeply interconnected. Eating living, raw foods is a simple, natural expression of that awareness, not an end unto itself. Natalia Rose gets this, and pushes the limits of what is typically discussed in the raw food arena by bridging the latest scientific breakthroughs with the little understood truths about food and energy, and how they can be better used to effect healing on many levels—physical, emotional, and spiritual.

On an individual level, Natalia's message is thrilling and empowering since it lifts the veil of misguided notions about how and what to eat, and offers the reader a key to a radically improved life experience. But she also offers a bigger message of universal healing, which will occur as more and more people successfully revitalize their energy fields using the recommendations she lays out in this book. While *Raw Food Life Force Energy* functions as a highly effective diet, it also seeks to uplift and unite humankind and all living things.

Deeply analyzed yet simply explained, this book will show you that detoxifying and rebuilding your mind and body in 21 days is something that anyone can do, regardless of the condition of your health and mind-set today. This book is not only for raw foodists, but also for those who simply want to cleanse out their system or transition away from the foods that are destroying their health and happiness.

In a world rife with modern illnesses and ill-functioning immune systems, Natalia offers us a fresh, magical solution—that of healing our bodies and minds through the very energy that we are made of. You will be delighted by how easy and pleasurable her 21-day program is to follow! Enjoy the delicious, natural recipes, learn the importance of food combining, and enjoy a healthier, new you. Create a free-flowing internal system and liberate your body from blockages that have developed from years of eating addictive foods. You'll find relief from stress, sadness, and anger. Natalia's words will inspire you to set a game plan that will help awaken you to your divine body and purpose. This in turn, my friends, will make our experience on this planet brighter and more powerfully united in light and love.

Raw Food Life Force Energy is so much more than another diet book. It is truly a beacon of light in the realm of raw food. Natalia's words are a warm breeze for the heart and soul. In a blissful blend of eastern wisdom and western science, her formula emphasizes compassion for the human temple so we can grow closer to our true nature—which is lean, healthy, energized, and divinely connected.

We are One.

All is Love.

Viktoras Kulvinskas is fondly known as the father and pioneer of the raw food lifestyle. In addition to cofounding the famous Hippocrates Health Institute in West Palm Beach, Florida, he has penned innumerable articles and five books on raw foods, including *Survival into the Twenty-first Century*, which has been dubbed the "Raw Food Bible" and the "Das Kapital" of the modern raw food movement by *SPIN* magazine.

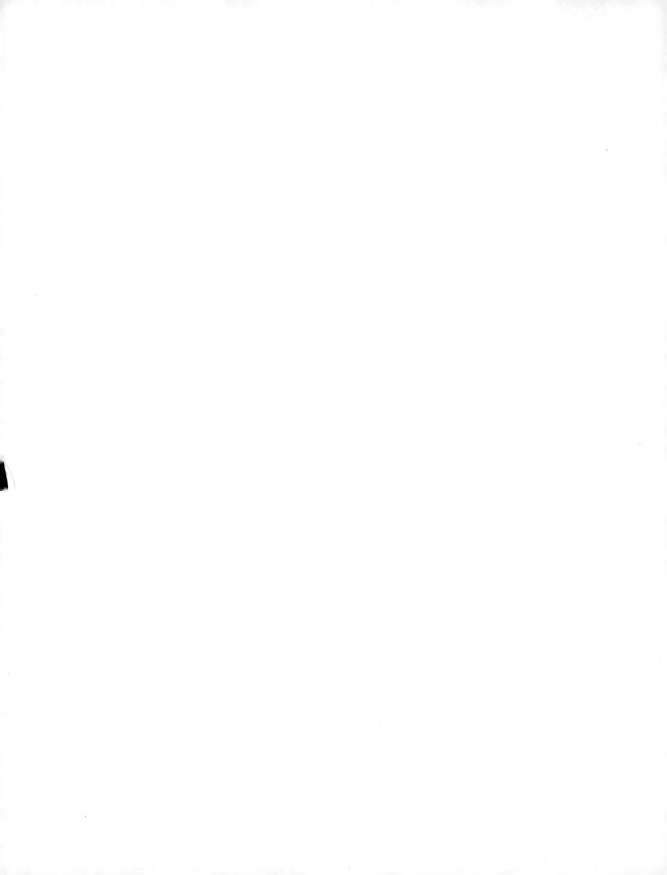

A MATTER OF LIGHT AND ENERGY

YOUR BEAUTIFUL, LEAN, ENERGIZED BODY STARTS RIGHT HERE

I know how you want to look and feel. I've counseled people from every walk of life and—whether they are actresses, homemakers, teachers, students, bankers, or socialites—they all want the same things: an energetic, glowing body; clear, youthful skin; and taut, toned limbs. They want to wake up in the morning aglow with energy and look in the mirror to find a face that looks rested and luminous *before* applying cosmetics. But it doesn't stop there; they also want to feel peaceful inside—inexplicably happy just to be alive. Does this sound like what you're looking for too? But does it sometimes seem like you're the only one who is going through life feeling groggy and weighed down? Do you fear that you'll never be able to achieve your desired weight or stop your body from deteriorating? Do you wish you could get beyond obsessing about how you look and feel in order to be a productive person? It is not too much to ask for. In fact, it's more achievable than you realize.

This book is going to introduce you to a whole new way of harnessing energy that will create a more attractive appearance, a much healthier body, and a radically improved state of being. First, I'm going to tell you all about this energy and how to get it. Then I will give you a totally comprehensive program that's easy to implement, which will completely rebuild your body.

For three weeks, make a small commitment each day to this program, and you can change the shape of your body and the shape of your life!

STEP INTO THE LIGHT

Energy has become such a catchall term that we have lost touch with its real meaning, along with the truth about how to energize our bodies. There is so much confusion about how to become more energetic and youthful, largely because so many competing products and supplements on the market today claim to be the answer to chronic lethargy and aging skin, offering nothing more than empty promises. Once you read this book you will never be tempted by these false promises again and you will understand why our modern ideas of getting energy from products such as sports drinks and energy bars are so foolish.

For many years I have counseled people on how to use food to cleanse their bodies, lose their excess weight, and improve their health. On a physical level, they have successfully removed obstructions within the digestive system and cells, making them thinner and younger looking. But something else happens on an energetic level: they begin to experience unprecedented rushes of energy and bliss. What my clients learn when they start eating according to the raw food energy principles in this book is that the body reaches this state of inner ecstasy, not because of the particular vitamin, mineral, and caloric makeup of my diet, but because (a) the foods they are now eating contain a highly coveted "essence" called "Life Force Energy" (which you are about to learn all about) and (b) the way they are eating encourages the swift removal of decades of waste buildup within them, enabling even more abundant Life Force Energy to flow into every cell in their body.

Life Force Energy is what does the work of healing and beautifying. The approach of this program is simply to optimize the body's receptivity to the consistent and abundant flow of this powerful energy.

A NEW WAY TO PERCEIVE YOUR BODY

Did you know that you are made of *living light-energy*? In 1905, Albert Einstein created what is now the most famous equation in physics, $E = mc^2$. What this tells us is that all matter actually consists of different variations of vibratory light-energy patterns. All matter, *including your body*, is made up entirely of pulsating, living light-energy.

Here we are today, more than a hundred years since Einstein proposed his Theory of Relativity, and we still overlook our body's intimate and integral connection to light or energy. With all of our modern advances, we still treat our bodies as though they are merely dense, material constructs maintained by the constant intake of solid food. This approach has left our society laden with weight problems, physical illnesses, and emotional imbalances. A simple but fundamental shift in perception about the nature of energy can correct these imbalances!

Today, we are finally going to apply Einstein's gem of a theory to your lifestyle to help transform you into a being of exceptional beauty, vitality, and joy. You are about to learn that the body you live in is animated and maintained by what we call Life Force Energy. While far too vast, complex, and mysterious to pin down into a nice, neat definition, Life Force Energy is commonly referred to by energy healers and quantum physicists as the pure and intelligent source of all energy that animates our world. How "intelligent" we do not yet know. Much about this emerging science still remains a mystery. But both the ancient schools of thought and the cutting-edge scientists in this field agree that Life Force Energy is a living, conscious matrix that moves in distinct, deliberate patterns and has an active, measurable energetic field.[1]

When you increase the flow of this power in your body, you will naturally and quickly become much more energetic, healthy, lean, and joyful. Feel free to get excited because it is the best news around for anyone who wants a beautiful, glowing body and a healthy, happy life. Best of all, it is relatively easy to do and starts to work immediately!

LIFE FORCE ENERGY: THE WAVE OF THE FUTURE

Now that quantum physics has confirmed that the body is made up of waves of light-energy[2] and that we are more than mere material machines, we need to look at our source of sustenance differently. If the blueprint of our body reveals waves of electromagnetic activity underlying and determining the dense physical material, we must revise our lifestyle and sustenance to incorporate this new information—particularly in terms of how we feed and care for ourselves. To put it differently, *if we are made up of Life Force Energy, we need a diet fit for Life Force Energy bodies.*

All other approaches to eating, dieting, and wellness are limited because they flat out disregard the core element of our being. For example, how could unnatural foods with no Life Force Energy sustain your light-energy body—even if these foods are low in calories and fat grams? They can't. They just create barriers to your natural radiance and beauty.

---

[1] www.calphysics.org/zpe.html.

[2] According to Werner Heisenberg, who developed the Uncertainty Principle in 1927, quantum calculations show that we and our universe live and breathe in what amounts to a sea of motion—a quantum sea of light. Lynne McTaggart, *The Field: The Quest for the Secret Force of the Universe* (New York: HarperCollins, 2002), 21.

The good news is that our modern world is changing to make enlightened eating and living easier and more affordable. Fresh, organic juice bars are popping up in Minnesota, raw food restaurants are thriving in die-hard beef-eating Texas, and women across the country are sharing their favorite natural recipes. Even Wal-Mart is getting hip to this trend! This means that living according to the principles of *Raw Food Life Force Energy* is getting easier and more accessible every day. This is just the beginning of a great awakening. Unnatural foods, counting fat grams and calories, and fad diets are losing ground. A more natural approach to dieting has already been set in motion, and a greater awareness of the way our bodies thrive on Life Force Energy is the next wave.

You may wonder if your body is the exception and wonder how I can make these bold promises without ever having seen you. Well, although I may not have seen you in person, I do know you're surrounded by an energy source that you've probably been deprived of for way too long. Regardless of how poor your appearance may be, you can increase the flow of Life Force Energy and bring your natural beauty to the light. Not only have I seen clients morph from average looking to highly attractive, but I have also had the pleasure of watching illnesses subside and relationships heal—all because of the energy and joy that surges through their bodies as they adopt a more enlightened approach to health and diet.

Finally you will see just how simple the principles of the *Raw Food Life Force Energy* are, and how inexpensive it is to apply them to your lifestyle. In my previous book, *The Raw Food Detox Diet*, I debunk the myths that we must eat raw food exclusively, sticking to dense, dehydrated raw foods and spending hours soaking and sprouting nuts and seeds. Simple, effective, enjoyable, and minimally expensive techniques are my signature, and this book is no exception. In fact, while you will learn the most powerful argument for eating a diet high in raw foods in this book, you will also learn that the highest-quality cooked foods are an important part of your diet as well. I will show you how to balance your raw and cooked food intake for the very best results. I invite you into my kitchen and my office to share in my experience so you can finally know what to eat.

THE PHILOSOPHY OF THIS BOOK

- We are dynamic-energetic/vibrational beings intrinsically connected with a universal energy system from which we can access an endless supply of Life Force Energy.

- In order for us to experience a perfect body, true health, and consistent joy, we need to clean our bodies and return them to their natural, harmonious light-energy quotient.

- Once we enhance the flow of Life Force Energy within our bodies, we will experience ourselves, each other, and our lives very differently.

- Once we are clean internally, harmoniously flowing with Life Force Energy, we will be infinitely more attractive to others because we will be physically more beautiful, lean, kind, clear, joyful people of right purpose.

I would like to take this opportunity to clarify that I am not presenting myself as an expert in vibrational energy fields or as a trained scientist, though I have researched the subject and consulted extensively with scientists in this field. I am a nutritionist who has practiced these theories successfully for years, and now wish to share my discoveries with you.

THREE STEPS BEFORE STARTING

READY . . . Recognize that almost everything you've been told about health from the media and conventional diet books is not dependable. If they leave out Life Force Energy and the fundamental prerequisite for clean cells and tissues, they are of very little value.

SET . . . Realize that you are going to have to do things differently if you are going to enjoy a healthy, disease-free life in a truly beautiful body.

GO! Embrace the beauty, the vitality, and the unprecedented pleasures that await you!

WHAT TO EXPECT FROM RAW FOOD LIFE FORCE ENERGY

- Effortless, abundant weight loss

- Glowing skin

- Improvement and eventual elimination of acne, psoriasis, and eczema

- Improved skin and internal tissue quality (firmer, younger-looking skin—even face, neck, and breast tissue)

- Reduction and eventual elimination of visible cellulite

- Markedly increased energy

- Fewer colds and flus

- Improved muscle tone, strength, and endurance

- Improved sleep patterns

- Improved positive attitude and a calmer disposition

- Increased mental acuity, including a sharper memory and better ability to focus on specific tasks

- Natural, spontaneous healing throughout your body

HOW TO USE THIS BOOK

Whether you are coming to this book hoping for more energy, weight loss, or just some new recipes, I highly recommend reading this book in its designated order the first time. I've identified a series of principles, which I swear by, and each one builds on the other; taken together, they will give you all the information you need to understand how to transform your body.

Each principle comes with practical applications, which I encourage you to undertake as soon as you're ready. The principles are the core knowledge of Raw Food Life Force Energy, but the practical applications spotlighted in each chapter are the directions you need to undertake to effect change in your body. All of the practical applications are designed to trigger rapidly flowing Life Force Energy in your body.

If you are in a hurry to get started, feel free to fast-forward to the 21-day program. This program starts with a test to help you determine your current Life Force Energy quotient. This is followed by easy-to-follow menus with convenient food choices. When you follow this simple plan, you should see a noticeable change on all levels of your physical experience in a very short period.

Part III offers more than seventy-five mouthwatering Life Force Energy recipes including soups, dressings, salads, raw and cooked entrées, and seemingly sinful desserts that are actually delightfully healthy. Most of these recipes are very easy to prepare. They are designed to redefine the concept of "health food" and introduce your palate to a whole new level of enjoyment!

Once you are well acquainted with the program and practical applications, you can graduate to using this book in more of a reference and refresher capacity. Whenever you're ready to go deeper, pick up the book again and increase the intensity of each of the practical applications for even greater results! As you see, this is so much more than a mere diet. It is an education, a fresh perspective, a way of life.

Remember, this is not a race or a contest. Anyone who approaches the Raw Food Life Force Energy program that way will miss the whole point. This is a program that truly honors your spirit and your body. We leave behind the competitive mentality, the stresses and the fears of the old sadistic approaches to beauty and weight loss. Instead, we embrace and learn to harness the naturally powerful, healing Life Force Energy that will surprise you with its gentle effectiveness! Step out of the darkness and become enlightened—both literally and figuratively—with the power of Life Force Energy.

PART I

THE PRINCIPLES

TAPPING THE SECRET LAWS OF LIFE FORCE ENERGY

In ancient Chinese medicine it was named *chi*[1] or *qi*. The Japanese named it *ki*. In India it goes by the name *prana*. The Hawaiians call it *manna*, and the African Bushmen call it *boiling energy*. They all recognized the same timeless force that we in the West call *Life Force Energy*. All ancient traditions understand that Life Force Energy needs to flow freely and abundantly from the energy fields surrounding us into our physical body for physical, emotional, and spiritual well-being to be possible.

If Life Force Energy is the power that breathes life into everything that lives, it's not something that you want to go through life low on, though most people do. The one thing everyone is after—a great-looking, healthy appearance—can easily be attained simply by increasing the flow of this key ingredient in the body. *In a world constantly in search of the miracle food, there is simply nothing on the planet that is as good for you as Life Force Energy!*

---

[1]Translated literally from Chinese to English, *chi* means "breath." This breath is more than just air. It is air clarified by a particular spiritual light; it is the charged essence of life. Luk Chun Bond, *The First 16 Secrets of Chi* (Berkeley: Frog Ltd., 2001).

Life Force Energy is a real, measurable force that surrounds everything on our planet. The ancient traditions considered it to be highly nutritive[2]; they knew there was a much more powerful nourishing force at play than just solid foods. Now it is time for the Western world to give credit where credit is due—not to milk, grain, and beef, which rob us of our life force—but to *chi*, *ki* and *prana*, which provide it!

Before I go into how to get more Life Force Energy flowing through your body, let's take a quick look at *how* energy actually flows. Just like everything else on the planet, you possess an energetic field, which we'll call your *energy body* for the purposes of this book. Your energy body emanates all around you in all directions, extending out several feet. It carries vital, life-enhancing energy into your physical body from the pulsating energy in the Universal Energy Field (the energy phenomenon that permeates all space and connects all things to each other[3]) into your personal electromagnetic field. From your electromagnetic field, it enters into your physical body through invisible pathways called *meridians*, making critical deposits to energy centers in the physical body called *chakras* and to the organs connected with points, best known as *acupuncture points*. This is how the body constantly refreshes its energy supply, recharging each and every cell with enlivened health. When we live inharmoniously, this whole system falls completely out of balance, distorting how we look and feel.

Your energy body is a mirror of your physical body and vice versa; depending on how your energy body flows, it determines the shape of your body and the shape of your life. If it is flowing well, you will look and feel marvelous. If it is not, you will

---

[2]Richard Gerber M.D., *Vibrational Medicine: The #1 Handbook of Subtle-Energy Therapies* (Rochester: Bear & Company, 2001), 171.

[3]"The existence of the Zero Point Field implied that all matter in the universe was interconnected by waves, which are spread out through time and space and can carry on to infinity, tying one part of the universe to every other part. The idea of 'the Field' might just offer a scientific explanation for many metaphysical notions, such as the Chinese belief in the life force or *qi*, described in ancient texts as something akin to an energy field." Lynne McTaggart, *The Field: The Quest for the Secret Force of the Universe* (New York: HarperCollins, 2002).

look and feel crummy. If you look tired and sallow, it's because your energy body has stagnated. If you are cellulite-ridden with varicose veins, your energy body is not feeding you the vital force that would otherwise prevent that from ever happening. If you are overweight, sluggish, and irritable, so is your energy body.

The Universal Energy Field, Life Force Energy, and your energy body are invisible only because they are made up of rapidly pulsating light-waves that can't be seen by the untrained, naked eye. Your energy body is sustained not by vitamins, minerals, and glucose, but by the very Life Force Energy of which it is made. I know it's hard to conceive of something like an energy field having an effect on your weight or emotions, but each is a mirror of the other and you'll be blown away when you see the physical results that come from harmonizing your energy body!

If it's more energy we want, we need to start living in such a way that encourages the abundant flow of Life Force Energy and brings us into a state of natural harmony. In the following chapters, I introduce the four principles that will help you better understand the characteristics of Life Force Energy so you can maximize its power in your body.

THE VIBRATION PRINCIPLE

"He who knows the Law of Vibrations knows all."

—HERMES TRISMEGISTUS, FATHER OF HERMETICS

Life Force Energy has a distinct vibration that will uplift, purify, rejuvenate, and energize every cell in your body, dramatically transforming your appearance and mind-set.

Matter is 99 percent space. Emerging from that space is vibrating energy. Everything that exists, be it natural or synthetic, has a vibration, an electromagnetic charge, and a resulting field. The earth itself, the moon, trees, animals, even your dining room table, all have a specific vibratory pulse that not only affects their own being, but the energy of those around them. Things that have a lot of Life Force Energy vibrate at a much more rapid rate than things that have very little Life Force Energy. For example, a plant vibrates at a much more rapid rate than a table. An apple vibrates at a much faster rate than a serving of fries. Human beings are designed to have a relatively high vibration (according to vibration specialist, Bruce Tainio, ideally somewhere between 60 and 80 megahertz).

If we fill our high-vibration body with low Life Force Energy substances, our natural vibration will slow down, effectively distorting and slowing the human energy pulse. Instead of progressing into healthier, more beautiful beings, we are digressing into inferior versions of ourselves. In this way, modern living, which includes the widespread consumption of low-vibration, low–Life Force Energy foods and drinks, fails to honor our natural design as individuals and as a species. This, of course, extends to all areas of our lives, from our health to our relationships, to our creativity, our leadership abilities, and so on.

DON'T BE DENSE

Low-vibration foods are typically dense (meaning they are low in water content), slow-vibing, and slow to move through the body. They include mainstream bread products, chips, cookies, and are most people's idea of a regular square meal. By contrast, high–Life Force Energy foods are "light filled," hydrating, and move rapidly through the body. In this way the concept of "light eating" takes on a whole different meaning. Light is a form of energy and vice versa. High–Life Force Energy foods are full of light—much of which comes directly from the sun. Every time we choose to eat white flour and processed foods instead of fresh fruits and vegetables, we take one more step away from our intended *lightness* and move toward an unnatural, unhealthy state of *denseness* as our vibrations mutate into ever lower frequencies.

We must focus on quickening the oscillations of our physical-energy bodies by taking in more light-filled, high-vibration substances and taking in less dense, low-vibration ones. Again, this will not only trigger physical healing, but will also help to correct the emotional imbalances that come with the frustrations of living in a dense, sluggish body.

PRACTICAL APPLICATION 1: CONSUME HIGH-LIFE FORCE ENERGY FOODS

Eating well is one of the quickest, easiest, and most fun ways to improve our vibrations. The foods that we consume daily can either rapidly deplete or invigorate us. The old adage "You are what you eat" should be revised to "You vibrate what you eat." A steady diet of low, inharmoniously vibrating foods will throw your entire energy body out of whack. Processed, refined, and synthetic foods are also unfit for human consumption because they completely deplete the *physical* body. This happens for two major reasons: (1) they are extremely difficult (in some cases, impossible) to break down and thus remain in our bodies, occupying previously clean, healthy cells; and (2) the chemical reactions that take place as these substances struggle to move through our bloodstream and intestines make us grumpy, bloated, and exhausted. This kind of lifestyle is a fast-track deathtrap because, meal after meal, it consistently removes our Life Force Energy, sneaking in dark lifelessness where light, beauty, and energy should be!

RAW PLANT LIFE—A TREASURE TROVE OF LIFE FORCE ENERGY

The highest-vibration Life Force Energy foods are those grown closest to the sun, such as tree fruits. Green vegetables, which contain synthesized sunlight in the form of chlorophyll, are the next most Life Force–rich foods available. But all edible plant life is a powerhouse of the most desirable Life Force Energy and will cause this element in you to skyrocket! Plants absorb the powerful Life Force Energy from the sun and the fresh, clean air. So by consuming plants, you are bringing that powerful energy into your energy field, thereby raising your body's vibrations. Anyone for a bowl of sunshine?

HARMONIOUS VIBRATIONS VS. INHARMONIOUS VIBRATIONS

As you read on, you will learn how to determine which high-vibration foods are harmonious with the human vibration and how to best incorporate less-than-ideal foods when desired. If you are interested in the approximate vibrational measurements for various foods, I offer a list at the end of the book on page 253, but the following Hierarchy of Life Force Energy Substances will be more useful, as vibrational measurements don't always tell the whole story. For example, some animal flesh registers fairly high when measured in megahertz against some other natural foods, but dead animal flesh is not harmonious with the human vibration. Anything that dramatically alters the state of a food substance, such as canning, freezing, pesticides, and cooking, will also affect the rate and harmony of its natural vibration.

The following list will give you a clear sense of which foods are ideal for human consumption and offer great amounts of Life Force Energy, and which are detrimental to your vibrational pulse and Life Force Energy flow. Until you reawaken your own innate ability to determine which foods are harmonious with the human vibration and contribute more life energy than they take, just refer to this list.

THE HIERARCHY OF HIGH-VIBRATION LIFE FORCE ENERGY SUBSTANCES

Highest Harmoniously Vibrating Substances

Sunlight

Fresh air and pure, clean water

Freshly extracted juices made from the highest-quality raw fruits and
vegetables

Organic sun-ripened raw fresh fruit (preferably but not exclusively organic)

Raw green vegetable life, including sea vegetation

Raw vegetables of all kinds, grown in nutritionally balanced soil

Raw honey

Medium Harmoniously Vibrating Foods

Cooked vegetables, including root vegetables

Raw organic nuts and seeds

Raw organic goat or sheep dairy products

Raw sprouted grains

Organic unsweetened dried fruits

Stevia, pure maple syrup, agave nectar, raw cane sugar

Low Harmoniously Vibrating Foods (perfectly acceptable through various stages of transition and helpful for many as staples even for the long term)

Cooked sprouted-grain products

Cooked grains

Other raw, organic dairy products (such as raw cow and buffalo dairy)

Free-range eggs

Organic, wild fish

Raw oils (cold or stone-pressed)

Interim Foods (while these items don't have the ideal harmonious vibrations or levels of Life Force Energy, they can be helpful as one transitions from a more common diet into this eating lifestyle)

Whole-grain products

Organic butter and cream (always choose butter over margarine or cooked oils; organic butter and cream are harmless in small amounts)

Organic nonraw cheeses

Free-range, grass-fed meats

Wine (fine in moderate amounts, as in one to two glasses a day, but not beneficial as commonly believed)

Inharmoniously Vibrating Foods and Elements (these have the most deleterious effects on the human physical/energy body)

Ordinary pasteurized cow milk, yogurt, and cheese

Infant formulas

Cigarettes

Hard liquor

Processed foods and synthetic ingredients

Mainstream animal fleshes (fish is the least detrimental flesh, followed by game, lamb, chicken, cow meat, and pork)

Pharmaceutical drugs

Technological radiation

X-ray radiation

DRINK IT IN!

Fresh fruit and vegetable juices are the most concentrated edible form of Life Force Energy available. When we juice fruits and vegetables in a juicer (not to be confused with a blender, which mixes instead of extracts), we separate the fiber from the critical energy of the plant, which is in its live enzymes, chlorophyll, and organic water. Remove the fiber and you remove the need to break down the juice; the liquid light energy goes straight to our bloodstream like an intravenous injection.

Without a doubt, consuming vegetable juices is the single most effective way to increase your Life Force Energy quotient through diet. They also taste delicious and refreshing, while delivering deep hydration and oxygen to the cells and bloodstream.

How do pharmaceutical drugs affect your vibratory energy and electromagnetic field?

As you could probably guess, they are damaging. Physicist and electromagnetic field expert Valerie Hunt calls them an affront to harmonious vibratory patterns. Hunt adds, in her book, *Infinite Mind* (Malibu, CA: Malibu Publishing Company, 1989): "[The experience of drugs] makes for an incoherent field with large quantities of very high and very low vibrations with no medium range frequencies. . . . Drugs do not help the evolutionary process, they hinder it."

Perhaps one day energy healing will become as popular as medication is today for chronic and acute physical symptoms, and we will be able to avoid much of the disturbance of these chemicals on the body's harmonious vibratory patterns. But if you currently take medication, this does not mean that you cannot still vastly improve your vibrational patterns. You can still dramatically improve your health and energy—and hopefully decrease and eventually eliminate the need for medication in time, depending on the severity of your condition. As always, be sure to consult with your doctor before making any decisions about your medications.

On page 158 I offer my most powerful vegetable juice recipe, Life Force Power-ade, which is also an integral part of the 21-day program on page 115.

Whether you opt to frequent your local organic juice bar or make it yourself at home, juicing fresh vegetables (particularly green, leafy vegetables brimming with chlorophyll) can energize every cell in your body. Many of my clients report that the vegetable juices alone have changed their lives!

WHAT ABOUT BOTTLED BEVERAGES?

Soda, coffee, and pasteurized juice drinks (juices that have been heated for preservation and bottled) *do not* generate Life Force Energy in the body; they deplete it. Like other inharmoniously vibrating substances, they rob the body of its own life force and pollute our inner pathways with carbon dioxide, chlorinated water, caramel coloring, fake and refined sugars, and aluminum (in the case of canned beverages).

Anytime you damage the structure of water, as in the case of these beverages, it cannot properly hydrate the body. These beverages are heavily marketed and consumed in the Western world for their supposed energizing properties, when in reality they ultimately dehydrate the body and deplete it of energy. Are you thirsting for something better? Raw, fresh-pressed juices (particularly fresh, organic vegetable juices that include some leafy greens) and fresh, pure water are high on the Life Force Energy spectrum and helpful in raising vibrations (see the elixirs in the recipe section for ideas).

A BAD CASE OF CONSUMPTION

When I walk into a mainstream grocery store, I cannot help but remark on how little in the store is actually food. I'm not referring to the paper goods and cleaning products, but the actual items that are billed as food. The aisles and aisles of food items are in no way fit for human consumption. Think: fluorescent orange, processed cheese slices; heavily processed luncheon meat mini-meals for kids; micro-wave fast food snacks, meals, and sauces; fluorescent-colored yogurt-snacks that contain so much food coloring they could double as paint; instant soups with ingredients that read like a radioactive experiment gone berserk; and packaged breakfast meats and sandwiches that guarantee heartburn before 8 A.M.!

These foods are successfully marketed as key parts of a balanced, normal diet lifestyle. Alien as they sound on paper, they constitute an entirely "normal" way of eating for millions of people. It's also normal to be sick, tired, and depressed all the time. It's as though consumers have become robots, buying and eating exactly what the commercials tell them to. I hope this book helps to snap some people back to their senses. These foods are not fun or healthy or in any way even remotely benign. They are killers! Killers of your cells, your joy, your beauty, and your physical independence.

It should be clear to you now that if you eat and drink foods of a low, inharmonious frequency, you cannot expect to avoid illness or function optimally. When it becomes a daily habit, your body and mind quickly degenerate. If the human body vibrates at between sixty and eighty megahertz, it makes sense that it should consume mostly fresh foods and water that have an energy frequency of at least sixty to eighty megahertz (which happens to be the natural vibration of properly grown and harvested fresh fruits and vegetables).[1] Foods that are processed outside the laws of nature are simply not harmonious with the human body.

To maintain our naturally intended, harmonious, high-vibration bodies, we should eat a diet of natural food. Yet, what is commonly termed *food* and worse still *healthy food* in today's mainstream market is far from nourishing or healthy. Viktoras Kulvinskas put it perfectly in his book, *Survival in the Twenty-first Century* (Woodstock Valley, CT: Omangod Press, 1975):

---

[1] These measurements are derived from Bruce Tainio's research, which employs the Tainio Technology Frequency Monitoring Device. See the Hierarchy of Vibrational Nutrition chart in the appendix.

Although Americans are eating more . . . they are receiving less nourishment. Real food, for the most part, is virtually unknown. Most Americans don't care. Their attachment to food is emotional and induced by advertisement. They load their shopping carts with a variety of colorful, unnutritious, plastic foods, saturated with synthetic ingredients. "Oh! But it tastes too good," they exclaim as they endlessly cram their stomachs, but remain unsatisfied.

Diet products, by the way, are among the worst offenders on the market! All the diet bars, "energy" bars; low-fat, low-cal, and low-carb products; protein powders; whey protein; sugar-free yogurts; one-calorie sodas; and "diet" frozen dinners (I could go on and on) are akin to slow-killing *poisons*! I'm not kidding. These synthetically manufactured foods and their cheap, processed ingredients (colors, chemical sweeteners, milk solids, white flour, etc.) are pouring disharmony and incoherent patterns into your body and your life, sabotaging any possibility of your looking or feeling your best. Fortunately, this old-school approach to dieting is nearing its end. Dieters are disillusioned and hungering for a better way.

Now that we know that the vast majority of processed foods from the multibillion-dollar health and diet market are in fact damaging to the human body, we may conclude that counting calories, fat grams, and carbohydrate grams has been the wrong emphasis for determining the health and weight loss benefits of foods. Are you finally ready to let go of these useless, silly measuring sticks once and for all, and accept that there is much more to health, vitality, and weight loss than calories, carbs, and fat grams? I understand it may be a reach for you if you've been dieting this way all your life, but take the leap—you'll finally get what you've been looking for!

Nearly all of my clients start out clinging to the calorie/fat gram model and fearing carbs, but those who have ultimately succeeded in transforming their bodies no longer give the slightest consideration to those things today. The harmonious Life Force Energy value of a food is the only information you will ever need to determine whether a food is healthy and conducive to weight loss. You need only consider the ingredients and chemical processes of foods to know how they measure up.

Many of you were probably surprised to hear about the 2006 study conducted by the *Journal of the American Medical Association*, which announced that a low-fat diet had no impact on the rates of breast cancer, colon cancer, heart attacks, and strokes. The American Cancer Society has called this $415 million federal study involving nearly 49,000 women ages fifty to seventy-nine over the course of eight years "the Rolls Royce of medical studies." Dr. Jules Hirsch, physician-in-chief emeritus at Rockefeller University in New York City, who has spent a lifetime studying the effects of diets on weight and health, called it "revolutionary" and added that it "should put a stop to this era of thinking that we have all the information we need to change the whole national diet and make everybody healthy."[2]

Clearly, a low-fat diet alone is not enough to prevent disease nor does it lead to vibrant health. Why is this? Because a low-fat diet can consist of low–Life Force Energy food. Foods that are generally recognized as low-fat, such as commercial yogurts, grain cereals, soy products, and so on, are all *dead* foods. On the flip side, you could positively thrive on a diet of high-fat avocados, raw nuts, cold-pressed oils, and fresh coconut coupled with calorie-rich fresh and dried fruits because you would be eating *live*, high-vibration food!

Vegans and vegetarians are not immune to misguided eating either, as most vegans and vegetarians consume just as many dense, inharmoniously vibrating foods as their standard American diet counterparts, just without the animal products. Meat is often replaced with even more damaging, highly mucus-forming, soy-based imitation meats and milks and dense, low-vibration, starchy meals and snacks such as white pastas and ordinary flour- and sugar-based baked goods.

Today there is a new movement afoot that recognizes the value of simple, fresh,

---

[2]Gina Kolata, "Study Finds Low-Fat Diet Won't Stop Cancer or Heart Disease," *The New York Times*, February 7, 2006.

straight-from-nature foods and a clean bodily system. This is the simple secret to a healthy diet, but it's so gimmick-free that our society is not wired to catch on without a great big strobe spotlighting it.

WHAT ARE YOU TUNING INTO . . .
AND WHAT'S TUNING INTO YOU?

One of the intriguing things about vibrational patterns is that they will both seek out and attract similarly vibrating patterns *and* they will tune other nearby vibrational patterns into their own patterns. You may have heard it said that "like attracts like." This also applies to our vibrations.

According to Dr. Valerie Hunt in her groundbreaking book, *Infinite Mind*, everyone has a unique energy field signature, like a fingerprint. Dr. Hunt's experiments conducted at UCLA suggest that, in addition to matter and thoughts, smells are also organized patterns of energy—that's what our olfactory senses pick up on when we are drawn to, or put off, by a particular scent. One hypothetical conclusion I've drawn from this idea is that the pheromones we give off—which appear to be so key to the romantic "chemistry" between people—may be directly linked to the organized energy around us. In other words, I believe we are attracted to a person's electromagnetic field, not just to the pheromones that emanate from it. Therefore, I propose that by changing our electromagnetic patterns through the lifestyle choices suggested in this book, we will emit a more attractive energy!

Consider, as the great artist, architect, and scientist Walter Russell suggests, that man is a product of "the electrical pattern to which he had attuned himself."[3] If you attune yourself to a more harmonious pattern, then your body, life, and experience will produce something entirely different and much improved! To *realize* the

---

[3]Quote by Walter Russell as recorded in *The Man Who Tapped the Secrets of the Universe* by Glenn Clark (Swannanoa, VA: The University of Science and Philosophy, 1946), 46.

upward potential of mankind by raising our vibratory energy patterns is the crucial first step that you must take. And you can start doing this just by eating high-vibration, sun-enriched foods!

I have seen many of my single clients transform so dramatically in body and spirit that they not only attracted a much higher-caliber mate but they also desired mates who were totally different from what they were seeking previously! It's as if a reorganization of their energy field fingerprints have made them mutually more attractive to other highly attractive people.

POINTS TO REMEMBER

- Food that is fit for human consumption is natural and fresh.

- Natural, fresh food has harmonic vibrations that are very high in Life Force Energy.

- While flesh would fall into the "natural" category, it carries the vibration of death and fear so it does not count as a harmoniously vibrating food. (It is not, however, the mission of this book to push vegetarianism. You can still make excellent progress by consuming some animal flesh while eating on the superior end of the high-vibration food spectrum.)

- If you like to eat fish regularly, there is definitely room for that, but try to cut back on chicken and red meat as much as possible. However, when cutting back on any kind of food that you love, take your time and don't feel pressured into making that change before you're really ready. Otherwise, you will develop emotional and psychological hang-ups, which will undermine your efforts.

- When you embrace a largely high-vibration, raw, sun-food diet, you will reach states of physical and energetic ecstasy.

- All people are designed to be high-vibration beings. Therefore, we must live in such a way that increases and maintains our naturally intended vibratory rate or we will devolve.

- If we deviate out of the range of harmonious vibrations, we set the stage for depression and illness.

- You may include low-vibration natural foods in this diet, but you should avoid the foods of incoherent vibration entirely, if possible.

- According to the Law of Vibrational Attraction, we attract the same energetic pattern as that which we vibrate. Therefore, the higher and more harmonious our vibrations, the more favorable the experiences we attract—in love, money, family relationships, and so on. Vibrate joy, attract joy! Vibrate beauty, attract beauty!

- Practical Application 1: Consume high–Life Force Energy foods.

THE FREE-FLOW PRINCIPLE

"Vitality Equals Pressure Minus Obstruction (V = P – O)."

—ARNOLD EHRET, *THE MUCUSLESS DIET HEALING SYSTEM*

In order for Life Force Energy to transform you, it needs to flow as rapidly and freely as possible through your body.

Now that you know how to increase the harmonious vibrations in your body through eating high-vibration foods, it's time to learn how to remove the obstructions that prevent optimal Life Force Energy from flowing through your body like a swiftly running river. The ultimate goal here is to create a body that operates in a state of *unobstructed flow*. Your body cannot become depleted when fresh Life Force Energy is consistently flowing through it. You might say that if Life Force Energy is the fountain of youth, the Free-Flow Principle is what gets you into that fountain.

The modern body is a body rife with obstructions. There are many reasons for this, but the top three are:

1. **FOOD WASTES:** The most obvious obstruction is in the form of food wastes that have not been eliminated from the body. Foods that move through the body slowly and are difficult to digest leave too much waste matter behind, creating all kinds of blockages throughout the body.

2. **STRESS:** Everyday tension, dispassionate living, financial anxieties, and/or relationship anxieties all create lactic acid buildup in the joints, which crystallizes and can be broken down only by a skilled massage therapist, hot Epsom salt baths, deep stretching, and a change of mental direction.

3. **EMOTIONAL PAIN, ANGER, AND RESENTMENT** create obstructions in numerous ways. They block the flow of our energy field and overwork our nervous system and adrenal glands by sending out excessive amounts of cortisol and adrenaline, which in large amounts are toxic. Pain and anger ultimately create restrictions in blood vessels around the heart, contribute to shallow breathing, and bathe the body in acidity, slowing and acidifying the digestion of all foods.

If you recognize yourself in any or all of the above points, you're not alone. Nearly everyone we know lives in a deeply obstructed body and world. But once you're aware of your own obstructions, you can more easily remove them with a little attention to the upcoming practical applications. And when you do, your life will be enriched beyond measure.

When your Life Force Energy is blocked by obstructions such as mucoid matter (the icky-sticky mucus created from unfit foods), excess embedded wastes from food and pollution, and emotional blockages like fear and pain, your vitality is severely reduced. When such blockages are removed, your vitality greatly increases. How simple! This means that if you only take in foods that leave minimal to no waste residue or mucus and you remove the excess buildup of waste matter, you will experience heaps of vitality—life force, chi, prana, manna, whichever term you like best.

The root of most illnesses is stagnation of the body's pathways and impaction of waste matter in its cells and tissues. The great naturopath Arnold Ehret put it this way: "Every disease, no matter what name it is known by Medical Science, is constipation: a clogging up of the entire pipe system of the human body."[1] In other words, stagnation of the body's pathways creates a breeding ground for bacteria and viruses to thrive, triggering more complicated illnesses. We can ensure perfect health simply by maintaining clear-flowing internal pathways for Life Force Energy, which will feed and nourish your physical body, making you shine as though you are lit from within!

Imagine it this way: if your finger has a piece of glass or metal lodged in it, it's going to be a painful breeding ground for an infection. That's exactly what's happening to your body on a larger scale. When your body is stuck with matter that doesn't belong there, physical, emotional, and energetic imbalances are bound to occur throughout your entire system. The solution is quite simple: remove the offensive object (the waste matter obstructing your inner terrains) and you'll be whole again. But don't wait!

If you are sluggish, tired, and irritable all the time, you now know that you're just obstructed and not getting enough fresh-flowing Life Force Energy. A clean, clear body feels like it rides on the wings of angels. I've experienced both extremes, and the sense of out-of-this-world vitality that I get from living in an unobstructed body is all the fortune I'll ever need. When your cells oscillate true vitality, you'll feel like the wealthiest person alive!

And here's the best part: you don't have to buy Life Force Energy—in fact, you *can't* buy it. No amount of money, vitamins, minerals, protein shakes, powders,

---

[1] Arnold Ehret, *Mucusless Diet Healing System* (Ardsley, NY: Ehret Literature Publishing Co., 1953).

creams, hormones, or B$_{12}$ shots are going to make you vibrant. Are you ready to learn how to remove the obstructions to this all-powerful energy in your body?

PRACTICAL APPLICATION 2: ELIMINATE THE FOOD WASTES FROM YOUR BODY VIA COLON HYDRATION, BODY BRUSHING, ALKALINITY, PROBIOTICS, AND SWEATING

Since we cannot get optimal Life Force Energy flowing through a body impacted with waste matter, I suggest my proven two-pronged strategy: (1) remove the waste that has already settled in our body, and (2) prevent new waste from accumulating.

Even though you may already be committed to eating high–Life Force Energy foods, you probably have several decades or more of waste from unfit consumption caked into your cells and tissues. Removing the waste matter from your body is clinically known as *detoxification*—that is, when waste matter is removed from the cells and makes a complete exit through the eliminative organs: skin, colon, lungs, spleen, liver, or lymph fluid/regions. Detoxification takes place in the human body continually from birth throughout its life.

WASTE = WEIGHT

Every time I explain to my clients that Waste = Weight, the light bulb immediately goes on. It makes both intuitive and common sense to them. This simple equation simplifies something that has baffled people for a long time. Waste matter in the body creates both disease and excess weight. If you are overweight and trying to lose it, don't kid yourself into thinking that your extra *weight* is not directly connected to the *waste material* that has overburdened your body's cells and tissues. It is!

The average person eats three to five meals each day (breakfast, lunch, dinner, and a couple of snacks) and that is considered typical and healthy. Our society places a great deal of emphasis on taking in adequate quantities of food without considering the importance of removing the waste matter that is consequently left behind. Listen up—if food is going into your body, once your body absorbs its nutritive value, the fiber and residual material need to come out. Otherwise, waste matter will pile up in your bowel, day after day, decade after decade, and whatever does not make it out bakes into your cells and tissues. I'm not suggesting that you should be able to have three to five bowel movements every day. On the contrary, even the healthiest colon could not be expected to keep up with the quantities of food intake typical of modern eating. No one wants to face it, but the fact is we eat way too much. Now, I'm not suggesting that you deprive yourself of hearty quantities if you desire them. I just want you to be clear that waste matter, if not removed in some way, is going to compromise the flow of your Life Force Energy. Decades of this buildup and the daily intake of food need to be cleared out.

PARDON ME, BUT I THINK YOU MAY HAVE MISSED A SPOT

We all know that if we go for long periods of time without showering or bathing or washing our clothes, our bodies will start to smell. In fact, our society is so concerned about cleanliness and smelling good that people use all kinds of antibacterial soaps, perfumed products, and abrasive detergents on a daily basis. And yet, few people pause to consider that a body will never be truly clean or smell good if it has a sluggish, overburdened waste management system.

Body odor is not a surface problem to be treated with skin products alone. Rather, it comes from the inside and is released through the skin, lymph exits, and mouth. If the interior of our bodies goes "unwashed" for long periods of time, the accumulation of putrefying material will breed a stench that no amount of soap or deodorant can remove.

Just as we bathe every day, wear clean clothes, and brush our teeth, we must also tend to the cleanliness of our insides day in and day out.

A NEW "MOVEMENT"

How can we wash ourselves internally? By a very simple procedure called colon hydration (a colonic or enema). This literally means that water enters your colon in order to help remove the buildup. A properly administered colonic is safe, easy, and, for the most part, comfortable. My colonic method of choice (there are several methods) is the "Gravity Method," which means that only the pressure of natural gravity is used to move the water. This is extremely gentle and safe, and there are many well-trained gravity-method colon therapists across the country.

While many people are excited by the idea of having a colonic, there are still many others who are concerned about the procedure, the expense, or just the very idea of it. If you are among the skeptical, I would strongly encourage you to reconsider. Even if you can boast of a healthy digestive system, you can be sure that your body is not passing everything you are eating. Consider the accumulation of waste over the course of your entire life, and you'll start to get a picture of the waste that your body swims in every day.

Contrary to what you might guess, the more high-vibration, sun-filled food you eat, the more you may need the help of colon cleansing. This food is so light filled it cleanses deeply, awakening sleeping poisons—which, of course, is the whole point. But you must be careful to loosen only as many toxins as your body is able to eliminate in any given time. Detoxification without colonics can result in symptoms such as headaches, pimples, sweats, sore throats, and so on. Colonics can help you avoid the discomforts of expelling the old poisons.

If for some reason you are still adamantly set against having a colonic, be very careful not to take in a diet of more than 60 percent raw foods. If you do, you may have great results for a couple of weeks as your body releases the waste that is sitting in your bowels now, drop lots of weight, and feel much more energetic. But unless you are very young or come from generations of pure, natural living, you will eventually start to have symptoms. If or when they do occur, it is a sure sign that your system is overloaded and only a colonic or enema will help. If you approach this cleaner way of living slowly, you will be far less likely to overload your intestines. Either dive into this diet lifestyle with gusto and incorporate some colonics as you need them, or go slowly to ensure a smooth transition.

As you may discover, with some exceptions, allopathic doctors do not generally encourage colonics. In my experience, they "pooh-pooh" them because they either (1) do not believe it's necessary and mistakenly think the bowel keeps up with the elimination of modern meals, (2) believe colonics will create a sluggish colon, or (3) are not familiar with the processes and, therefore, are not aware of the benefits. To the first point, we know that the bowel cannot keep up with junk foods, unfit foods that compound upon themselves while dehydrating in the colon at 98.6°F. To the second point, the only things that create a sluggish colon are these same unfit foods, caked-in waste matter, and the habitual consumption of laxatives. These are the culprits that make it necessary for gastroenterologists and surgeons to amputate whole sections of the digestive tract.

Can we pretend there is no irony in the fact that some of the very same doctors who are "anti-colonic" get enthusiastically behind truly extreme and damaging procedures like stomach stapling and gastric bypass surgery? As you may be aware, these highly invasive and life-altering procedures are currently the most popular treatments for morbid obesity. Tragically, many merely overweight people rely on them as a way to trim down.

I want people to know that there is another option—nutritional cleansing and internal bathing—to bring overweight people back to a healthier size rapidly without any of the devastating consequences of gastric bypass surgery. In my experience, colleagues and clients who have long been dedicated to nutritionally cleansing their body with the support of colonics experience consistently strong peristalsis (the wavelike muscular contractions of the intestines), thorough elimination, vibrant health, and perfect weight. What's more, they all look and feel far younger than their years!

To their credit, many forward-thinking allopathic doctors are supportive of colonics—particularly the rapidly growing niche of medical doctors who see the importance of melding traditional medicine with holistic healing, or integrative medicine. I believe that procedures such as colonics will only gain in popularity over the next decade. Until then, it will serve you well to educate yourself and always get more than one opinion as you plan your personal health strategy.

If you are concerned about the expense or finding someone near you or you just want to take it slowly, you can find an excellent, simple enema kit for at-home use as well as a list of recommended colon therapists in the United States and abroad on my website: www.TheRawFoodDetoxDiet.com.

DRY BRUSHING

Dry brushing is one of the greatest detoxification tools after colonics. Dry brushing is done with a special natural-bristle body brush that you can find in any health food store. The brush costs only about $7 and is one of the cheapest, most effective

Check Out Your Tissue Quality

Take a look at your largest organ—your skin. The quality of your skin will give you an idea of the quality of your organ tissues. When you put something unnatural into your body, imagine it going straight into your tissues and organs. How can your skin and eyes glow if your tissue quality is laden with junk? When you put only natural, fresh foods into your body, your tissue quality will reflect that and you will glow with the radiance nature intended. When your skin is getting oxygenated from within due to excellent blood flow and unobstructed pathways, the signs of aging and cellulite can be reduced dramatically without any expensive creams or plastic surgery.

beauty and health treatments you can enjoy. When you dry brush your body correctly:

- Your lymphatic system is stimulated to push out wastes.

- The dead skin is removed, making way for your skin to breathe fresh oxygen into the tissues for greater oxygenation throughout.

- Lactic acid and other lymph waste is brushed away.

- Cellulite is targeted and diminished.

- You are left feeling totally energized.

How to Dry Brush Your Body

Stand in your bathtub, shower, or anywhere you are comfortable, completely dry and nude. Take the dry brush off the long wooden handle. Since you should always brush the body in upward strokes toward the heart, with the exception of the torso, begin brushing the tops of your feet in firm strokes toward the ankles. Then make firm strokes up the calves, toward the knees (make two strokes over each spot). Brush upward along the backs of the knees, the groin, and the armpits (these are the major lymphatic drainage regions, so pay extra attention to them). Next, brush the fronts of the thighs from the knees to the groin and hip sockets and the backs of the thighs in firm upward strokes. If you are prone to cellulite or "saddle bags," spend a moment brushing those areas in a circular motion. Next, brush the torso in downward strokes; then brush the palms of the hands well from the fingertips to the wrists—followed by long brush strokes from the wrists to the armpits and shoulders. Be sure to brush equally on both sides of the body. Finally, place the brush back on the wooden stick and brush as much of your back as you are able to reach. This whole process should only take about three to five minutes. A new brush can feel harsh the first couple of times but will quickly soften, so brush more gently at the beginning if you need to. This practice will leave your physical and energy bodies completely refreshed and invigorated!

HELLO PROBIOTICS!

A strong colon has lots of healthy bacteria, or good intestinal "flora," which helps to move waste out at maximum efficiency. Plenty of this healthy flora protects against the overgrowth of the bad bacteria that commonly develop as putrefactive wastes sit in the lower bowel. Ample good bacteria easily fends off bad bacteria. A healthy intestine has a bacterial balance ratio of approximately 85 percent good bacteria to 15 percent bad bacteria. The average Westerner, however, has a bacterial balance that is the *reverse* of that! What will happen if you have more bad guys than good guys? The bad guys will win. Have the bad guys won the fight for your intestines? Do you have irritable bowel syndrome (IBS), bloating, gas, constipation? If so, they have.

It's time to strike back, overcome the bad guys, and help the good guys get in there and reclaim your intestinal territory. Think of it as a "war of the worlds" in miniature! All you need is the right probiotic. Probiotics are the healthy bacteria (the good guys). However, regular probiotic supplements are killed by the stomach acids long before arriving in the intestines, where they are so desperately needed. Recently, the Japanese have formulated a specially protected pill in the form of mini-pearls that work very well. I recommend taking one or two every day on an empty stomach. You'll feel it at work pretty quickly in the form of increased bowel movements and less gas and distention. You can order them from www.therawfooddetoxdiet.com.

Food Sources of Probiotics

Cultured, fermented vegetables like kimchi and pickles are beneficial for the intestines only if they are consumed within four days of preparation. Beyond that, the concoction develops high levels of lactic acid and should be avoided.

Many people herald yogurt as a superfood because natural yogurts contain healthy bacteria. The problem is that the milk protein in mainstream yogurt makes it so hard to digest that any benefits gleaned from the probiotics are not worth it (not to mention that most yogurts are full of coloring, sugar, and aspartame). One big exception to this rule is *raw goat* yogurt and kefir, a cultured goat milk product. Because they come from unpasteurized goat products, the protein is easily digested. Some states allow dairies to produce and sell raw dairy products, while other states have strict laws against it. Despite the fact that raw dairy products are not popular today, they were the only form of dairy products available before we started shopping in supermarkets. If you are getting your raw products from a reputable raw dairy, there is nothing to worry about (although pregnant women should still take the precaution of avoiding raw dairy on the off chance of contamination).

Properly raised and packaged raw dairy is—forgive the expression—a completely different animal than pasteurized dairy. In fact, raw goat cheese is one of the major staples in my, and my family's, diet. I particularly recommend the Alta Dena Raw Dairy's cheddar-style goat cheese, which I enjoy in surprisingly abundant amounts with no physical drawbacks—great news for cheese lovers! If you can get raw dairy products (particularly raw goat and sheep products) try them; you will be delighted with the effect of the good bacteria from raw goat yogurt and kefir entering your intestinal tract. The trick with the raw goat yogurt and kefir is to (1) swish them around in your mouth and predigest them with your saliva and (2) take them on an empty stomach so that they do not mix with any other food. I've found them to be most effective when taken in two- to four-ounce servings, two to three hours prior to dinner.

Another option is to drink the juice of freshly pressed Jerusalem artichokes and cabbage. This must be consumed immediately, as the cabbage oxidizes rapidly. Drink six to twelve ounces a day on an empty stomach for a week to boost your healthy bacterial flora.

Bruce Tainio, an agriculture technologist, vibrational field expert, and the founder of Tainio Technologies, shared with me a compelling insight into the nature of pests and bacteria that sheds a lot of light on the human intestinal bacteria balance. "Nature," he explained, "sends these things out to a sick or injured living thing to get it out of the gene pool." He pointed out that nutritionally balanced soil and plants do not have pests and therefore do not need pesticides. "It was not until modern farming took hold and the farmers were not knowledgeable about how to create nutritionally sound soil that pesticides became necessary." Tainio often experiments with the nutritional contents of plant soil in his laboratory gardens. For example, he'll deliberately create an imbalance and watch as the beetles appear in greater quantities, then he'll correct the soil and they will disappear.

First, consider how this simple correction in the soil could eradicate the need for pesticides. Now, consider how this simple correction in the cleanliness and nutrition stability of our internal terrains could swiftly eradicate the need for antibiotics. A great many of my clients who were slaves to antibiotics in the past have found that they they no longer need them at all, since adopting the high-vibration raw lifestyle. Once we achieve a healthy intestinal balance, we no longer suffer from destructive bacteria and parasites.

ALKALINE FOODS CAN MAGNETIZE UNFIT FOODS AND WASTE RIGHT OUT OF THE BODY!

The benefits of a highly alkaline diet are well known in health circles and have been the focus of numerous health books. This is because our blood pH is naturally alkaline (7.4). If we eat too many acid-forming foods, we will throw our blood pH into an overly acidic state, which is devastating to the whole system. But the other reason that alkaline-forming foods are so helpful is that they actually help to magnetize waste matter out of the cells.

You may be familiar with the term *polarity*. Everything in creation has polarity, and in atoms it can be observed in the form of a positive (+)/negative (−) charge. At the subatomic level, the proton is the positive-charge particle and the electron is the negative-charge particle. Unfit foods that are acid forming carry a positive charge. (Note that in this context, "positive" is bad, and "negative" is good.) Acid-forming foods that carry this undesirable positive charge reduce the levels of desirable negatively charged energy in our body! Acid-forming foods also set the stage for the development of highly acidic, putrefactive waste matter, which we want to avoid at all costs. The overwhelming positive charge multiplies, creates congestion, and prevents oxygen from flowing effectively for vibrant health and well being. Once cells are clogged with too much acidic material, the body begins to suffocate and one's Life Force Energy grows consistently weaker.

On the other hand, raw fruits and vegetables and their juices, fresh air, and sunlight carry a negative charge. As you know, in the case of magnets, a negative charge and a positive charge attract each other. In the case of acid waste residue, alkaline-forming foods, with their negative charge, will magnetically attach to the acidic wastes and literally pull them into the eliminative channels for release.[2]

By the same token, we can also decrease the negative charge that keeps us healthy by being exposed to too many positively charged ions in our environment. If we are "rightly charged" (negatively/alkaline charged) and then start eating acidic foods and spending time indoors under fluorescent lighting, in front of computer screens, and in a sea of wireless technology, we will compromise this ideal magnetic charge.

If you must be in an office or an acidic environment all day, there are still some things you can do to help remedy the compromising effects:

1. Get out in the fresh air and sunshine as often as possible throughout the day.

2. Breathe deeply to oxygenate and rebalance your energy regularly.

---

2. While this has yet to be scientifically proven, the scientists I've consulted with all agreed that this is a perfectly logical hypothesis that clearly seems to work in the body.

3. Enliven your body through yoga, dance, and massage (but don't *over*exercise since that can cause lactic acid to acidify blood as well).

4. Transition into the best alkaline-forming diet you can.

5. Keep negative emotions in check to keep acidic, incoherent vibrations at bay.

I am realistic and understand that many people coming to this program are living in big cities, working in offices, and struggling with various stresses. This is completely typical. I don't expect you to change your lifestyle all at once. Just change what you can, as soon as you can. Changing your diet is the most manageable, logical, and effective first step to take. The rest will come in time. It's even okay (though obviously not ideal) to keep working with your technological gadgets and swim a bit in the wireless sea if you can counter these acidic charges with plenty of alkalinity. But you cannot possibly expect to live, eat, work, and internalize acidity in every aspect of your life and have any degree of health, well-being, or Life Force Energy. So think about what you can realistically change, and adjust your lifestyle accordingly.

Not everything that is alkaline has a negative charge. There are some exceptions, such as calcium, sodium, and potassium. Although they are alkaline minerals and alkaline forming in the body, they happen to be positively charged. Likewise, some alkaline-forming foods, such as citrus fruits, are acidic in nature but leave an alkaline "ash" in the body and are therefore considered alkaline forming, highly beneficial foods! By the same token, some alkaline elements, such as milk and meat, are actually highly acid forming in the body and ultimately very detrimental.

DISTINGUISHING BETWEEN ACID-FORMING AND ALKALINE-FORMING FOODS

If you stick to the idea of eating harmoniously vibrating foods you will naturally eat a high-alkaline diet. In fact, notice how the Hierarchy of High-Vibration Life Force Energy Substances on page 22 is virtually identical to the list of alkaline/acid foods and elements below:

Highly Alkaline

Sunlight

Fresh mountain air

Fresh green vegetable juice

Other raw vegetable and fruit juices

Raw vegetables

Sprouts of all kinds

Neutral (enjoy daily if desired)

All cooked vegetables

Cooked roots and starch vegetables

Highest-quality grains such as millet, quinoa, amaranth, spelt, and kamut

Low Acid (perfectly acceptable on a regular basis)

Sprouted-grain breads and other whole, unrefined grains

Raw milk products

High Acid (avoid)

Artificial foods

Food additives

Nicotine/smoke

Drugs

Sodas

How do the environment and technology contribute to the acid charge of our physical and energetic bodies?

You may be surprised to know just how much your natural beauty and the harmony of your vibrational energy body are compromised by the modern world. As anyone who's ever been in the Rocky Mountains or experienced the feel of the early morning surf can tell you, it just feels better there. It feels deeply refreshing, energizing, and healing to be in a natural, unpolluted place on the planet. There is an electromagnetic reason for this: pure air gives off a negative ionic charge that both harmonizes with our own being and pulls out the impurities within us so we actually feel better.

Of course, we cannot all pack up and move to these ideal spots on the globe. Most of us center our lives in and around cities, where we all too frequently complain of feeling tired, lethargic, moody, or simply off-kilter. This should come as no surprise, for the human body is designed to live in a fresh, rightly charged environment. Now, imagine you are standing in front of a television or computer screen. That screen is giving off (+) charged ions. These ions will literally jump onto you and *stick* to your healthy (–) charged cells, reducing the overall (–) charge of your body.

This constant onslaught of positive ions triggers physical symptoms as well. Headaches, for example, are a very common symptom of sitting in a wrongly charged office all day. Once one goes outside into the rightly charged fresh air, one usually feels better immediately. Chronic fatigue and colds are also common symptoms. If you are swimming in an acidic pool all day, your immune system is going to be severely compromised.

There are some objects that are *believed* to help combat the effects of the technological ions, such as Planet Tachyon's magnetic devices, which claim to neutralize radiation (hydrogen peroxide is known to do this as well). Crystals have been used for this purpose too.

A Battery of Stress

The rush of worry, fear, and shock associated with stress causes free radicals, which carry tremendous acidity, to run rampant through our bodies. Acidity weakens the organs and the conductivity of energy in the body. A healthy, unobstructed body will recover from a temporary state of stress, but a body weak in Life Force Energy could easily "overdose" on negative emotions. If the body is so deeply impacted with waste and awash in acidity, any further stress could put one over the edge in the form of a heart attack, a stroke, an ulcer, and so on. In order to correct this and enable yourself to recover quickly from a major stress, you need to have adequate alkaline reserves. You get these reserves from eating high-vibration, natural raw foods and immersing yourself in joyful activities.

Laughter is a great alkalinizer! The well-known *Saturday Review* writer Norman Cousins alkalinized himself back to health through laughter by watching *Candid Camera* and Marx Brothers movies. Perhaps Shakespeare put it best in *The Taming of the Shrew*: "And frame your mind to mirth and merriment, which bars a thousand harms and lengthens life."

Master colon therapist Gil Jacobs spoke to this in one of our conversations: "Keeping a positive attitude is not so much about what's in your head, it's literally what's in your cells. You need to be relaxed, calm, and happy on the physical plane because if you have constant worry, pain, and sadness, you are triggering poison into your bloodstream on a chronic basis. This is also why people who try to cure illnesses with health foods alone don't always heal."

All these techniques aside, the best way to combat the overcharging effects of the technological world is by eating a steady diet rich in high-vibration, raw, unadulterated foods, and by eliminating waste matter from our bodies through colonics, body brushing, deep breathing, and sweating. Given the direction of our technological world, I believe that the standard American bathroom will eventually include the following features to counteract the detrimental positive charge of the environment:

Infrared sauna

Colonic unit

Natural-bristle body brush

Chi machine (a device that moves the body in a way that optimizes its
  flow of chi or Life Force Energy)

PRACTICAL APPLICATION 3: PUMP LIFE FORCE ENERGY THROUGH THE BODY WITH THE LIFE FORCE ENERGY POWER BREATH

Remember oxygen? It is one of the greatest sources of Life Force Energy. It's always there for the taking, but few of us actually take more than a fraction of our capacity of oxygen into the body. Yes, we are breathing all the time, but the average breath is shockingly shallow. It's as if we've all become too lazy to breathe.

The typical Westerner only breathes as far as the upper portion of the lungs. The lungs are like giant balloons that can be filled to extraordinary capacity. When very deep breaths are taken, two major things happen: (1) Life Force Energy floods the body, oxygenating and enlivening the whole being, and (2) the force of the oxygen helps to push through obstructions in the body. Deep breathing creates an internal pump for the body—think of your lungs as a chi machine keeping everything circulating. One of the things that attracted me to deep breathing is that when you do it properly, your organs actually get

a massage! When your breathing lacks power, your circulation slows down and everything stagnates.

Since we cannot live for even a few minutes without oxygen, it's no surprise that shallow breathing leads to premature aging and even premature death.

THE LIFE FORCE ENERGY POWER BREATH

Learning how to breathe properly is essential. It's funny, babies do it perfectly, but by the time we become adults we lose touch with this incredibly simple, utterly critical part of our human design. The Life Force Energy Power Breath feels like an exaggerated inhale and exhale, but it is necessary to exaggerate it in this way in order to hasten the intake of oxygen and repattern your automatic breathing throughout the day. Practice the following steps as often as you can and reap the benefits of increased oxygen flow throughout your physical and energy bodies:

Step 1: Sit comfortably and begin to inhale through the nose sending the air straight down into the belly. If you place your hand on your belly, you should notice your hand is pushed out by the expansion of the belly. Imagine you are trying to inflate it as much as possible. Inhale for a count of four full seconds. It will feel like you are inhaling beyond what feels typical for you, and then beyond that, and then when you think you really must exhale, inhale even a drop more and hold for a moment.

Step 2: Now, for the exhale: This will also last for a count of four full seconds. Deflate yourself completely through your nose. It's a strange, exaggerated sensation if you've never done it before. Exhale fully and before inhaling again empty the remnant air even more thoroughly (still through your nose) as you draw your belly into your spine as far as possible.

Repeat the above two steps at least three times and begin to feel the peaceful, highly charged vibrations dance throughout your body. Inflate deeply. Deflate deeply. Inflate.

Deflate. Let that deep, rhythmical cadence fill you with fresh oxygen and energy, and then expel the old breath to take in even more fresh air.

Breathing this way is like building a fire in your body. The more oxygen you take in, the brighter and bigger the fire can burn! This is an exercise you can do anytime and anywhere to flood you with Life Force Energy, help remove mental and emotional blockages, and raise your vibrations.

OXYGEN = EXERCISE

The only reason formal exercise is considered necessary today is because we are a sedentary culture; we move very little and eat lots of low-vibration, acidifying foods that clog the body and block the flow of oxygen. When you remove the obstructions in the body through deep breathing, detoxification, and ideal eating, you won't even need rigorous exercise because you will be getting all the vital life force that you need right into your cells naturally.

Don't get me wrong, I'm in no way knocking rigorous exercise as a lifestyle choice. The endorphin rush or runner's high that you hear about—that's absolutely real and it's triggered by the increased oxygenation that comes from breathing deeply as a result of intense physical exertion, and it definitely has a strong impact on the flow of Life Force Energy. However, you certainly don't *have* to approach physical movement in this manner for it to be maximally effective.

For many years before I lived according to the Raw Food Life Force Energy diet, I depended on exercise to keep my weight and mood stable. I always felt better after exercising because I was oxygenating my body. But even with all the intensity of my workouts, I never felt as euphoric, light, and energized as I do now, even when I am at my most inactive.

Arnold Erhet, in his book *The Mucusless Diet Healing System*, went as far as to say that the lungs, not the heart, are the body's essential "pump," since the heart could not function without the lungs pumping oxygen. Oxygen is the prerequisite for our lives and contains highly concentrated amounts of Life Force Energy. Still breathing?

PRACTICAL APPLICATION 4: ENLIVEN YOUR BODY

I have long felt that the term *exercise* connotes something you might not want to do but have to do. Further, such concepts as "pounding the pavement," "hitting the gym," and "pushing weights" are just more high-stress extensions of our demanding lives. I prefer an approach that focuses on "enlivening" the body—a renewing experience that takes us out of our day-to-day madness and leaves us feeling uplifted, connected, and whole. Enlivening the body requires shaking up the stale energy to create a huge increase in your body's ability to flex and circulate Life Force Energy! Think of dancers and yogis, whose bodies move fluidly without resistance or rigidity.

What's important is that Life Force Energy flows unobstructed throughout your body—not that you burn X number of calories, run X number of miles, or that you're in the "fat-burning zone." The goal is to bring your body back to a lean *fluidity* that cannot be achieved through standard aerobics, weight lifting, or the neon numbers on gym equipment. In my private practice, many people who come to me work out every day, often with a trainer, and are still overweight. The modern approach to exercise can only go so far—and that's not nearly far enough!

Like Life Force Energy, fluidity cannot be bought. Yet fluidity (which is synonymous with such terms as *flowing, flexible, lithe,* and *agile*) is the trump card of health. *Any* body, regardless of age, is capable of achieving a youthful leanness, energy, and fluidity through a gentle, conscious transition. Yoga, dance, and Tai Chi are the best ways I know of to create maximum total body enlivening!

THE TWENTY-FIRST CENTURY YOGI

Yoga, when done properly, is a powerful way to enliven and totally rebalance your body. It also helps firm and slim your body. Most important, yoga helps to create a flexible spine, which ensures the constant flow of Life Force Energy between the physical and energy bodies (the spine is the pathway of the Kundalini, which is the pathway that feeds the chakra system and the meridians). Yogis define youth by the flexibility of the spine, not by the number of years one has lived.

A yogi recently mentioned to me that, in her experience, a person's physical flexibility was directly connected to his or her flexibility in other areas of life. Keep this in mind as you work on becoming more fluid in all areas of your life.

If you are used to modern exercise, you may not realize that yoga is deeply challenging and demanding. A good yoga practice will have you sweating and strengthening muscles you never knew you had. However, the goal of yoga is not to develop a "rock-hard body," but to develop a level of physical strength and mental awareness that enables us to hold challenging postures with grace, and release tensions and stresses in the body. I give yoga my highest endorsement. Find a good class and learn from a skilled teacher who has a good understanding of alignment and you will see how beautiful and strong your body can be! You don't have to do it for a specific amount of time. Even ten minutes of "sun salutations" (the core yoga warm up) several times a week would be sufficient. It doesn't take much to generate dramatic results on all levels.

TAI CHI FOR LIFE FORCE ENERGY

Tai Chi is one of the oldest and most effective methods of enlivening the body and improving the flow of Life Force Energy (or "chi"). You may have passed by a group of people in the park doing what appears to be a funny dance in slow motion. This funny dance is actually a powerful exercise that looks deceptively easy. Those who practice Tai Chi know differently. The exercises start to work immediately to connect them with the source of Life Force Energy and healing. Many Tai Chi exercises are specifically targeted for weight loss (such as "drawing the moon") and youthful appearance (such as "lifting the sky"). There is even one for breast enhancement ("separating the water")! For a great comprehensive book on Tai Chi that includes all of these exercises and more, I recommend *The Art of Chi Kung: Making the Most of Your Vital Energy* by Kiew Kit Wong (New York: Cosmos Publishing, 1993).

SHAKE, STOMP, AND MOVE THE ENERGY WITHIN YOU

Not only is dancing fun and a great opportunity to listen to your favorite music, but you can move the way you want to move, while releasing old energy and refreshing your body with new energy. You can do it in short bursts for as long as you want. Duration, like calories, is a poor measuring stick. If in two minutes you can shake up the old energy and feel your body become incredibly loose and free, then that's all the time you need. If you're really enjoying it, then keep going. Get out of the "duration" headspace and just let yourself move without rigidity or inhibition.

The trick to energizing your body is to be as utterly spontaneous as possible and let loose when the moment or the music moves you. If you approach physical movement in this way, you will not look at it as a chore, which can derail this process. You will be able to express yourself with natural, un-self-conscious joy. You will be more in tune with how your body wants to move, which is inherently healing and cleansing. And finally, will be able to release the physical and emotional tensions of the day.

In addition to yoga and dance, massage is highly effective at increasing fluidity, releasing internal blockages, and thereby increasing the flow of Life Force Energy. Massage is not an indulgence; it's a necessity. In fact, more and more health plans are covering massage therapy, particularly for those with chronic and degenerative health issues. Find a good therapist and go as often as your budget will allow. It will make a tremendous difference to your fluidity and energy levels. To those of you who claim not to have the time to care for yourself in these ways, I say you don't have time *not* to, and if you don't, you'll probably have even less time still on this planet!

FOOD FOR THOUGHT

I have one last thought to leave you with on the idea of free-flowing vitality, and it comes from Walter Russell in his book, *The Man Who Tapped the Secrets of the Universe* (Wayneshoro, VA: The University of Science and Philosophy). When he was asked if he ever gets tired, he replied:

> Can energy tire or become fatigued? Certainly not, for all energy is the thought-energy of the universal Creative Force, and that never lessens. The universal intelligence is constant and forever balanced. What is it then that makes us say we are tired? Only one thing: an unbalanced body, nothing more. If we think we are tired or ill, it is only because we have done something to unbalance the bodily conductivity of the universal electric current which motivates it. . . . An inner joyousness, amounting to ecstasy, is the normal condition of the genius mind. Any lack of that joyousness develops body destroying toxins. That inner ecstasy of the mind is the secret fountain of perpetual youth and strength in any man. He who finds it finds omnipotence and omniscience. I therefore say to you that tiredness and fatigue are effects caused by ignorance of Nature and disobedience to her inexorable law.

POINTS TO REMEMBER

- Every person's vitality is directly linked to the flow of Life Force Energy in his or her body. When Life Force Energy flows within without obstruction, the ordinary individual becomes extraordinary.

- Increasing oxygen flow is one of the best ways to increase fresh Life Force Energy in and around us.

- In order for Life Force Energy to flow, we must remove the obstructions in our body through foods that collect waste matter by maintaining a clean, healthy colon and opening the body through yoga, dance, and massage.

- A diet high in alkaline foods and harmoniously vibrating foods (which are basically one and the same) will prevent new waste matter from building up in the system and allow Life Force Energy to flow continuously, offering the greatest levels of vitality!

- Don't forget to look out for the hidden acidifying elements in your immediate environment and avoid them—or at the very least neutralize them by increasing the alkalinity around you with alkaline-charged foods, fresh air, and sunlight.

- Use the power breath and raw foods to move as much oxygen through the body as possible.

- Yoga and dance are essential for enlivening the body and creating the kind of flexibility and fluidity the body needs to maximize its flow of Life Force Energy.

A REVIEW OF THE PRACTICAL APPLICATIONS THUS FAR

Practical Application 1: Consume high–Life Force Energy foods.

Practical Application 2: Eliminate the food wastes from your body via colonics, body brushing, probiotics, alkalinity, and sweating.

Practical Application 3: Pump Life Force Energy through the body with the Life Force Energy Power Breath.

Practical Application 4: Enliven your body.

THE QUICK-EXIT PRINCIPLE

If we eat wrongly, no doctor can cure us; if we eat rightly,
no doctor is needed.

—DR. VICTOR G. ROCINE, NORWEGIAN PHYSICIAN, CIRCA 1930

The foods and combinations of foods you eat must make a
quick exit in order for them to contribute to your Life Force
Energy quotient.

You have already learned a lot about how to maximize your Life Force Energy
through high-vibration foods and improving your internal flow. Grasping and applying the Quick-Exit Principle is the final step.

Before we go further, note that this principle is perfect for those looking for
quick weight loss results without doing anything else. It is very typical for people to
shed weight quickly after only several days of "quick-exit" eating.

The Quick-Exit Principle tells us that the most health-generating foods and
combinations of foods are those that enter the body, give the body what it needs, and

then get the bloomin' heck out of there! Hydrating fruits and veggies do exactly this, which makes them the quickest exit foods around.

What is the reasoning behind the Quick-Exit Principle? Whenever you eat a food or combination of foods that is difficult to digest, you paralyze the flow of Life Force Energy because "slow-exit" foods and meals use up the vital energy and enzymes that are working hard to break these substances down. This all amounts to a loss of energy that could have been put to many more supportive, anti-aging tasks within the body. If you eat a slow-exit meal once in a while, it's not a big deal because the body can afford the occasional energy leach as long as the meals do not pile up. But if you eat a heavy, slow-exit meal several times a day or week, the constant drain on the body's Life Force Energy, the expenditure of precious enzymes, and the pileup of waste multiplies, overtaxing and disfiguring the body.

Quick-exit foods and quick-exit combinations are the opposite of this—they are foods and combinations of foods that pass easily through the body and help correct this waste buildup issue very quickly and can correct many of these imbalances single-handedly! One of the major reasons that quick-exit foods and quick-exit combinations work, beyond the fact that they are less apt to leave behind waste matter, is that they require less energy to digest. They give us more Life Force Energy than they take.

If we are constantly exhausting our supply of energy breaking down slow-exit meals, we won't have energy for the things our body really needs to do like turn over new cells, heal organs, and drive us effortlessly through otherwise demanding lives.

This concept of quick-exit eating finally puts to bed the myth that food should "stick to your ribs" for long-lasting sustenance. The opposite is actually true. The longer a food remains inside you, the more energy that food will take from you. What will keep you going all day long are fresh fruits, vegetables, and vegetable juices that deliver maximum sunlight, oxygen, and Life Force Energy but don't stick around to weigh you down!

PRACTICAL APPLICATION 5: EAT "QUICK-EXIT" FOODS IN "QUICK-EXIT" COMBINATIONS

While the quickest-exit foods are also the highest–Life Force Energy foods, such as raw fruits and vegetables, you are not expected to live on these foods exclusively—that would be too extreme for most people. Any high-quality, minimally processed natural food, including fresh fish, whole-grain pasta, sprouted grain breads, raw goat cheese, and brown rice, can make a quick exit from the body if it is enjoyed in a quick-exit combination.

Let's take a look at how long some commonly eaten foods take to pass through the stomach: fresh fruit, when consumed alone on an empty stomach, leaves the stomach in about fifteen to twenty minutes. Vegetables take a little over one hour. A serving of pasta, a serving of whole-grain cereal, a filet of fish, or a breast of chicken spends about three to four hours in the stomach. Steak and other red meats take a little longer. If you were to eat chicken with some raw vegetables and steamed broccoli alone, it would still take only three to four hours because this would be a quick-exit combination. However, a more typical meal in our culture would be a combination of chicken with french fries or rice, or bread (as in the case of a chicken sandwich). When you mix foods in this way, the transit time of the meal skyrockets from approximately three to four hours in the stomach to approximately eight hours in the stomach, backing up the whole digestive system and exhausting your Life Force Energy. This happens every time foods are "miscombined," creating a slow-exit meal.

Quick-exit combinations are really very simple to create once you get the hang of it. Best of all, when you properly combine your quick-exit foods into quick-exit meals, you can eat as much as you want because your body is getting a significant break from all the time and energy that went toward digesting slow-exit combinations before. The body is so rested that it is able to throw off much more waste matter and start breaking down, and eliminating much of the old buildup in the body. This is why people typically lose weight very easily when they practice this application. Remember the equation Waste = Weight? You simply won't create or hold waste if the food you eat makes a quick exit.

Once you learn the simple, common-sense steps involved in creating quick-exit combinations, you'll find this way of eating extremely liberating because you can eat highly satisfying quantities of food without feeling drained or putting on weight!

QUICK-EXIT MAKEOVERS FOR SLOWER-EXIT FOODS

If you are just starting to transition away from a mainstream diet, simply give your favorite foods a quick-exit makeover. For example, while a steak combined with a potato spends eight to twelve hours in the stomach, a steak combined with a raw salad and steamed green vegetables spends only about four to five hours in the stomach. If it's pasta you're craving (ideally whole-grain pasta), just have it with marinara sauce, unlimited vegetables, and some raw vegetables, and it should leave the stomach in about three hours. You could even have a couple of whole-grain cookies for dessert, guilt free! Learn the simple rules for mixing foods in the chart below and you'll be on your way. If you were to choose only one Raw Food Energy principle for optimum digestion, energy, and weight loss, apply the principle of eating quick-exit combinations. Once you know what categories your favorite foods fall into, it is not at all difficult to combine your meals properly.

The Five Food Categories

1. Starches: breads, pastas, whole grains, potatoes, legumes, cooked corn, avocados*

---

*Avocado is technically a fruit. If eaten without other starches (just with raw vegetables), it will combine perfectly with all fruits, including dried fruits.

2. Fleshes: all animal flesh, eggs, and cheese

3. Nuts and seeds

4. Dried fruits

5. Fresh fruits

The Five Fundamental Rules of Quick-Exit Combining

1. Starches combine only with other starches and all raw and cooked vegetables.

2. Fleshes combine only with other fleshes, all raw vegetables, and all cooked nonstarch vegetables.

3. Nuts combine only with other nuts, seeds, dried fruits, bananas, and all raw vegetables.

4. Dried fruits combine only with other dried fruits, avocados, bananas, nuts, and all raw vegetables.

5. Fresh fruit should only be eaten alone on an empty stomach.

QUICK-EXIT COMBINATION TABLE

(Never mix any of these four categories with one another, with a few exceptions.)

STARCHES	FLESHES (FLESH-PROTEIN)	NUTS/SEEDS (FAT-PROTEIN)	FRESH FRUITS
Whole grain breads	Fish	Raw nuts	Citrus
Brown rice	Eggs	Raw seeds	Bananas (combine well with fresh as well as dried fruits)
Sweet potatoes	Chicken	Raw, unsulfured dried fruits (combine well with raw nuts/seeds but should otherwise only be enjoyed alone or with raw vegetables, always on an empty stomach)	
Avocados (technically a fruit but combines with starches and dried fruits)	Meat (beef, lamb, pork, etc.)		Plums
	Game		Nectarines
Legumes (lentils, cooked peas, beans, etc.)	Shellfish		Grapes
	Raw cheese (while it should ideally only be combined with vegetables, some people can get away with combining it with flesh)		Berries
Cooked corn (raw corn combines as a vegetable)		Mature coconut (small and brown)	Other fruits
Young coconut (large and green, or shaved; also combines with raw nuts/dried fruits)			
Pasta			

PRACTICAL APPLICATION 6: PRACTICE EATING "LIGHT TO HEAVY"

When my clients first come to see me, they are usually surprised when I tell them that the most important thing about breakfast is not to eat it. Common knowledge has it that breakfast should be the largest meal of the day and dinner should be the smallest. This misconception has deprived people of too many delicious, hearty dinners!

The rule of eating "light-to-heavy" asserts the opposite view: we should eat the lightest possible foods in the morning, and gradually increase the density of the foods we eat, so that the heaviest meal is dinner. You should begin in the morning with the lightest foods, meaning fresh raw juices and fruits. Then move on to slightly denser foods in the middle of the day, such as vegetables, nuts, dried fruits, and avocados. At the end of the day, have any flesh, cooked grain, cheese, and so on.

Yes, you read that correctly—dinner, not breakfast or lunch, but dinner should be the heaviest meal of the day. Before you get going about having the whole day to burn off calories, let me remind you that we've left calorie counting behind! Try it for one day and you will feel the difference in your energy

Keeping Yourself Fresh Through Quick-Exit Combining

If you're seeking the highest levels of vitality and weight loss, simply eating pure foods is not enough. If you mix raw nuts, fresh fruits, sprouted grains, juices, raw oats, and so on in the same meal, you might as well be eating fried chicken and mashed potatoes for all the work the body has to put into digesting that combination of foods. Moreover, ill-combined meals will create carbonic gas in your system. Carbonic gas is the noxious by-product of fruits and grains sitting on old matter in the body. It can make you bloated, eat away at your bones, and is a main cause of body odor!

level! Heavy foods in the daylight hours steal our energy and inhibit elimination. Follow this tenet, and you will see how your energy skyrockets and your eliminations improve!

The "light-to-heavy" concept also applies to the order of a stand-alone meal. Ideally, you should eat the lighter dishes/foods before the heavier ones. Have your salads and/or other raw foods before the cooked foods and starches or animal products. Now, if you're just starting to adopt the light-to-heavy principle, following it within the context of each meal is not as important as following it within the context of an entire day. Master the light-to-heavy order on a daily basis first, and then you can take it to the next level if you like.

By eating light to heavy, you are not making huge demands on your digestion at every meal. As the saying goes, "There is a time to laugh, a time to cry, a time to live, and a time to die." We do not do all these things at once—if we did, we'd be placed in an asylum. On a digestive level, there is a time to digest, a time to assimilate, and a time to eliminate. We cannot effectively do all three at the same time. When we eat dense food throughout the day, all three of these critical aspects of digestion are compromised. You'll be amazed by how much stronger your digestive process is when you give each phase the opportunity to do its job, uninterrupted. Your Life Force Energy flow will thank you for it!

Fish or Meat?

Fish is definitely the preferred choice among animal fleshes because it is much easier to break down and will, therefore, leave less waste residue and leach a lot less valuable Life Force Energy. Red meat, by contrast, creates a lot of extra work for the body and, by sitting in the body for so long (our intestinal tract is much longer than that of typical carnivores), negatively impacts the good bacterial balance of our intestines as it putrefies therein. But be careful to select the freshest wild and organic fish. Fish combines beautifully with all raw vegetables and low-starch, cooked vegetables.

Don't worry if you don't fully grasp the concepts of quick-exit combinations and light-to-heavy eating right away. The meals that are laid out in the 21-day program, coming up in Part II, are already properly combined and follow the light-to-heavy order, so you don't even have to think about it.

Quick-Exit Tip Sheet

- Fresh fruits should be enjoyed only on an empty stomach—either as the first thing to enter the body in the day or at least three hours after a properly combined meal. It should never be eaten as dessert or within eight hours of an ill-combined meal. Lemons and limes are the only neutral fruits that can be mixed with anything.

- Starches go with all other starches and vegetables—nothing else!

- Fleshes go with all other fleshes and cheeses (in most cases) and vegetables—nothing else.

- Nuts go with all dried fruits and raw vegetables—nothing else.

- Dried fruits go with all raw vegetables and raw nuts, and also go perfectly with avocados. Bananas are a dense fruit, so they can be combined as fresh fruit and dried fruit, which means they also go with avocados.

- Chocolate, almond milk, mustard, ketchup, spices, and all vinegars are neutral (though vinegar is acidic, so you may want to use it sparingly).

- Raw goat cheeses are the best form of cheese and go best with vegetables, but most people can get away with mixing them with flesh, too.

- Butter and cream go with everything except nuts, dried fruits, and fresh fruits.

IN WITH THE NEW

OUT WITH THE OLD

The quality of a food is determined by its ingredients and "sunlight quotient."

The quality of a food is determined by its amount of calories, carbs, and fat grams.

The healthiest foods make a quick exit.

Good foods stick to your ribs.

Keep meal combinations as simple as possible.

Mix starch and protein for a "good square meal."

Eat your heavy meal at the end of the day.

Eat your heavy meal in the morning.

Soy and peanuts are unfit foods.

Soy and peanuts are the best diet foods.

To increase your energy, take in raw foods and juices that provide Life Force Energy.

To increase your energy, eat dense power bars and protein shakes.

To keep slim, give your body breaks from digesting.

To keep thin, eat small meals frequently.

Dinner should be the heaviest meal of the day.

Breakfast should be the heaviest meal of the day.

Lasting youth can be yours free of charge.

Lasting youth is impossible, but you can age gracefully if you can afford lots of plastic surgery and expensive creams.

A REVIEW OF THE PRACTICAL APPLICATIONS THUS FAR

Practical Application 1: Consume high–Life Force Energy Foods.

Practical Application 2: Eliminate the food wastes from your body via colonics, body brushing, probiotics, alkalinity, and sweating.

Practical Application 3: Pump Life Force Energy through the body with the Life Force Energy Power Breath.

Practical Application 4: Enliven your body.

Practical Application 5: Eat "quick-exit" foods in "quick-exit" combinations.

Practical Application 6: Practice eating "light to heavy."

THE NATURAL BLISS PRINCIPLE

If I could bottle this up
I could make a million
I could sell everybody in town on what I've been feeling
'Cause it's guaranteed to put a smile on your face
A song in your heart after one little taste
Folks couldn't get enough
If I could bottle this up

—PAUL OVERSTREET, "IF I COULD BOTTLE THIS UP"

When your body is filled with free-flowing Life Force Energy,
you'll experience waves of natural bliss.

When the body is cleared of obstructions and flowing with Life Force Energy, you
will experience a sensation of complete joy and well-being that cannot be explained
by any outside experience or material phenomenon.

Can you remember the last time you were bursting with joy—not for any specific reason, just inexplicably blissful? Have you ever felt inexplicable joy flood your being without any effort or thought? If not, you have been seriously deprived! But you're not alone. Most people haven't a clue about this state of natural bliss that is everyone's birthright. No one told me about it either. In fact, it took me the better part of thirty years to make the connection, and I'm one of the lucky ones. Most people spend their lives chasing after money, public approval, and material possessions, without ever tapping their extraordinary, innate capacity for joy.

HAPPINESS IS OUR NATURALLY INTENDED STATE

With all due respect to those who have experienced deep suffering or hold fast to the belief that life is a constant struggle, I firmly believe that happiness is our natural state. When you live in a body flowing with abundant Life Force Energy, you are filled with a natural contentment.

When I asked a scientist friend of mine who had done extensive research on the African Bushmen—on what the Bushmen perceive to be the purpose of life—my friend replied, "the Bushmen believe that life is one great party and that we are here to enjoy it." Colonizers have called the Bushmen "savages," but they sound awfully civilized to me. Their outlook on life is heavily influenced by their intimate connection with nature.

Westerners today are so far removed from natural sources of energy, sustenance, and joy that we are inclined to believe that *depression* is normal. Joy is something extraordinary in our society—only a very few among us walk through life joyfully. Meanwhile, instead of pausing to consider the deeper implications of the widespread diagnosis of depression, we simply treat it with pharmaceutical drugs.

I believe that the root cause of depression can almost always be traced to abnormal living, eating, and spiritual unrest—and that correcting these imbalances of modern living will effectively eliminate depression. How often, though, do we propose dietary and lifestyle adjustments as a course of treatment for the disease of depression? How often do we educate those suffering from depression in our culture about the effect of unfit foods on our physical and emotional balance? Very rarely, if ever. Instead, we prescribe drugs and occasionally add some talk therapy to the mix. Although antidepressant drugs can be a valuable aid for those who are going through a time of intense stress or trauma and are struggling to transition back to a balanced life, the cultural norm of knee-jerk prescription writing is shameful.

Can we blame this practice on some sinister combination of ignorance, laziness, and monetary motivation? Are some people too lazy to make real changes in their lives, preferring to pop a pill? Perhaps that may be true in some cases. But in my experience of working with many clinically depressed clients, I have learned that the majority of them would prefer *not* to take medication if there is a way to avoid it. In fact, many of them list this as a key reason for coming to me to detox. Now, I'm in no way suggesting that everyone suffering from depression could be fully cured by the practical applications of the Raw Food Energy Diet—some mental illnesses and unfortunate life circumstances are far more dire and need much more support. But, in the case of the average depressed Westerner, there is a better way.

I hope you will go even one step further and look at the following practical applications as much more than a way out of depression. See them as a way *into* your natural inheritance: a lifetime of harmonious emotions and inexplicable bliss!

CRIMINAL CONSUMPTION

Is it possible that we all are addicted to illegal substances? Dare we consider that what is illegal according to the laws of nature are laws of a much higher standard than what is deemed illegal to the federal government? Is it an exaggeration to compare abstaining from unnatural refined foods to abstaining from drugs? Is it a stretch to say that the modern world breeds junkies who don't even know they are junkies, addicted to substances that make them crazy? If you want to learn just how crazy these mainstream foodstuffs can make you, I recommend that you read Carol

Simontacchi's *The Crazy Makers: How the Food Industry Is Destroying Our Brains and Harming our Children* (New York: Tarcher of Penguin-Putnam, 2000).

What if I go a step further and suggest that we are not only "users" but that we are criminals in the court of natural law, consuming illegal substances that will land us with a life sentence in prison. We are depriving ourselves of natural freedoms, subjecting ourselves to hopelessness and a seeming inability to lead the lives we want. Sure, we may be able to come and go as we wish, moving between towns, states, nations, and continents, free to buy, believe, or wear whatever we want. But what is all of that worth if we are imprisoned in an imbalanced, low-energy, diseased body? What is freedom if not freedom from illness, depression, fatigue, stress, and self-loathing?

LOVE AND FOOD: A MIND-NUMBING RELATIONSHIP

We need to learn to distinguish between the foods we love and the foods to which we are addicted. From childhood, we are conditioned by trusted adults to consume foods they deem healthy (from parents insisting we drink our milk to advertisers hypnotizing us with commercials that justify the everyday consumption of high-sugar cereals and other highly processed foods). These commercials and their subliminal messages send us mindlessly into the kitchen at every intermission for more chips and cookies. Couple this with the fact that every time we put a bite of food in our mouths we momentarily forget our worries, fears, and obligations.

It's very easy to see how food addiction can be confused with love. No matter what hurts, we can always register a pleasure response from our food "fix." At this point we find ways to justify eating these foods; we tell ourselves that our body needs and deserves them—that we should have what we "love." You are probably addicted to certain foods just as smokers are addicted to cigarettes. The first step, of course, is admitting that you may have a problem. The good news is that by simply avoiding these unnatural, processed foods for several days (eating the delicious Raw Food Life Force Energy versions of them instead as listed on page 153), you can start to overcomc and be liberated from these addictions forever. But as long as you keep eating them (which means the addictive substances are flowing through your bloodstream), you will remain addicted and those foods will be governing your life and your body instead of the other way around.

HOW YOUR CHAKRA SYSTEM INFLUENCES YOUR PHYSICAL AND EMOTIONAL EXPERIENCE

As we discussed earlier, ancient Chinese and Indian medicine identified the major points of energy in the body as the chakras. It has been further established that these unseen energy centers correspond to the endocrine glands. The endocrine glands are hormone manufacturers. It stands to reason that imbalances in certain chakras due to imbalances in the energy body would stimulate imbalanced hormone production from the corresponding glands. For example, if the throat chakra, which is the energetic center of communication, self-expression, and relationship with food (overeating, deprivation, and so on), is out of balance, it could manifest in thyroid imbalances in the form of either hypo- or hyper-thyroid issues.

The third-eye chakra which represents intuition, corresponds with the pineal gland which governs the production of melatonin and serotonin, and governs the circadian rhythms (sleep cycles). So if you are moody or experiencing episodes of insomnia, balancing your third-eye chakra (through harmonizing your energy body as a whole) should help correct it. The chakras must be nourished in order for their corresponding

Mood responses in children and adults are profoundly affected by diet and environment. Chemicals in food and environmental pollution have been shown to have a deleterious impact on the brain and neurological functions, leading to everything from attention deficit disorder to obsessive-compulsive disorder. It makes sense that foods that contribute to physical illness would contribute to mental and emotional imbalances as well.

organs and glands to be healthy. By the same logic, when unfit foods stimulate the glands to produce unbalanced levels of hormones, they in turn create imbalances in those corresponding chakras, and ultimately damage the energy body as a result.

PRACTICAL APPLICATION 7: REMOVE THE ENVIRONMENTAL OBSTACLES BETWEEN YOU AND YOUR NATURAL JOY

Now that you know that food wastes and inharmonious additives and food preparation methods are making you miserable, you're probably already envisioning the results of a diet that will reverse this and lead to greater joy. Great! That means you're ready to stop consuming the foods that are robbing you of your joy and start taking in more foods and meals that fill you with happiness. As you do this, notice how your moods shift and how your emotional load seems to lighten. Remember that the standard American diet goes by the acronym SAD in health circles. It really does make you sad!

To whatever extent you are ready, I also highly recommend removing the non-food environmental obstacles to your joy, such as the audio and visual stimulation in the form of magazines, television, and movies that degrade your thoughts with vulgarity, graphic imagery, gossip, and violence. Don't be afraid to try a media fast for a day, a week, or even a month—whatever would be a stretch for your media lifestyle. In a media fast, you eliminate as many of the following as possible: TV, magazines, newspapers, radio, and the Internet for a given period. Similarly, you might try a shopping fast. At least once a year, I undertake a "shopping strike" where, for one month, I buy only absolute necessities such as food and household cleaning equipment. It's not as hard as it sounds, once you commit to it. The most valuable reward is that you begin to see just how much you are "sold" every day. When you go off the strike, you become a much savvier buyer, much more in tune with what you actually need and desire, as opposed to what you *think* you need and desire!

Another environmental factor to be mindful of are your relationships. In toxic relationships, we put up walls between ourselves and others that keep us from giving and receiving love and harmonious vibrations. The fewer walls we put up, the more we send out good feelings to others, and the easier it is to love our fellow man. Think of your interactions as exchanges of Life Force Energy. Remember that consistent positive actions deliver consistent positive results. Refrain from gossip and speaking poorly of others. Focus on the best in people. Learn the art of forgiveness and be grateful for those who teach you lessons about yourself. This is a topic that truly deserves a whole book, and many very good ones have been written already. But in the meantime, the simple practice of gentleness and appreciation of your fellow man, friends, and family will enrich your life with joy and Life Force Energy.

PRACTICAL APPLICATION 8: NOTICE HOW MODERN THINKING AND LIVING LEACH YOUR NATURAL JOY

As the saying goes, "the beginning of fear is the end of power." Modern thinking, which is largely driven by the media, constantly sends us messages of what we should fear. When we are in a state of fear—of our finances, relationships, health, future, and so on—we shut down completely. It's not easy to overcome this deeply ingrained mental patterning and replace it with one rooted in confidence, but as you begin to select the thoughts and images you allow into your consciousness more carefully, you increase the flow of Life Force Energy, inspiration, and joy. Do not underestimate the power your own thoughts, and those of others, have over your life and energy flow.

Also remember that fear, anger, jealousy, and stress are highly acidic. Consistent exposure to these emotions and experiences are just as damaging to the body as an acid-forming substance you might eat, drink, or smoke. They will quickly rob you of your attractive charge, radiance, beauty, and youthfulness.

Therefore, try to build up reserves of love, compassion, and enthusiasm for the people and things you enjoy, and watch how these alkaline emotions contribute to a more radiant you.

FAST-FLOWING LIFE FORCE ENERGY CAN REVITALIZE YOUR WORK LIFE

One of the things you'll notice as you increase your Life Force Energy flow is how inspired you will become in your creative pursuits. To draw on the wisdom of Walter Russell again, in *The Man Who Tapped the Secrets of the Universe* he writes about joy as it pertains to modern work:

> If you have no joy or happiness in your work, finding it to be drudgery instead, you will fatigue from the devitalizing discharge of the energy . . . as the years go by, your mind becomes dull from its constant devitalizing draining of energy and the body disintegrates prematurely. . . . The greater the joy within one's inner-consciousness, the greater the force of the recharge of thought-energy within one; and that is why I have climaxed my defining words with the word ecstatic . . . by "ecstatic," I mean inner joyousness, and by inner joyousness I mean those inspirational fires which burn within the consciousness of great geniuses, fires which give to them an unconquerable vitality of spirit which breaks down all barriers as wheat bends before the wind. . . . the almost hidden joyousness of deeply banked fires which need dramatic expression to evidence their existence in work. This joyousness is that quiet, invisible boiling up of the inspired spirit of the great thinker.

Joy, inspiration, and great ideas are all interconnected and spring naturally from a clear-running river of Life Force Energy. We all carry within us the potential for brilliance and vitality, but if we want to enjoy it, we must start by removing the obstacles to our Life Force Energy!

EMBRACING A LIFETIME OF HIGH-VIBRATION RAW LIVING

"Look where you are going because you will inevitably go where you are looking."

—EMMET FOX, *FIND AND USE YOUR INNER POWER*

One of the questions I'm most frequently asked is: "Is this something you just do for a few weeks or a few months, or is it something you do forever?"

When most people hear the term *detox*, they usually assume that it is something one does for a short time—perhaps for a day or a week. They hardly ever consider that one would *live* that way. But logically speaking, ask yourself, *Does it really make sense to detox just to retox? Why would I ever want to revert to a lifestyle that has made me look and feel miserable in the past?* Sure, you may slip up and revert to your old ways for short periods (such as on vacation or when life throws you a curve), but the principles in this book are intended to comprise *a way of life*—and, in my experience, it's the happiest lifestyle imaginable!

If you embrace these principles and apply them faithfully to your diet and environment, you can occasionally afford to have less-than-ideal foods and experiences, because they will be neutralized by all the goodness that you're taking in the rest of the time.

When done right, the Raw Food Life Force Energy program will help you derive more pleasure from your life than ever before. Here's how:

- You will feel physically lighter after, and between, meals.

- You will enjoy the most delicious, rich, sweet, hearty natural foods on the planet.

- You will derive great pleasure from the way your body and complexion begin to look.

- Your new look and confidence will breed a natural feeling of empowerment.

- You will feel inspired and derive greater enjoyment from your natural talents and abilities.

- You will be less critical, resentful, and envious of others.

- You will experience inexplicable waves of bliss from the high vibrations running through you.

- You will enjoy greater mental acuity and think more quickly on your feet in your professional life.

- Your energy will skyrocket—physically, mentally, and spiritually.

PRACTICAL APPLICATION 9: LINK PLEASURE, CUSTOMIZATION, AND CONVENIENCE

A self-proclaimed gourmand myself, I have stuck with this lifestyle for as long as I have by celebrating my love of food at every meal. The proof is in the palate: food is flavorful; we are supposed to derive pleasure from eating. When you think of all the depths and dimensions of flavor in natural foods, you will see what a banquet awaits you in the natural world. Consider the depth of flavor in maple syrup compared to refined sugar, which is supersweet but otherwise flavorless. Think of the layers of spice and sweetness in a ripe peach or pear. The best part is that the best foods taste great and help keep you flowing with energy and joy.

One of the best things about this diet is that it includes all of your favorite tastes—fatty, acidic, sweet, salty, starchy, and so on—so you can always keep your palate happy. For example, when you want *salty* tastes, you may use sea salts or Nama Shoyu, a raw soy sauce. Regular soy sauce is okay, too, but as you progress you'll want to use the raw version.

When you want to add *sweetness*, you may use Stevia (I recommend the NuNaturals brand), agave nectar, pure maple syrup, organic dates, organic un-sulfured dried fruits, and raw honey.

If you crave a *cheesy* flavor, use the raw goat cheese. You'll be amazed at how good the Alta Dena cheddar-style raw goat cheese is! I also like the Shiloh Farms brand, and you may find others at your local markets, dairies, and food co-ops. Avoid all fake, processed cheeses such as the ones made from soy. Even the almond cheeses in the health food store are highly processed and filled with frightening ingredients. You can make your own seed and nut cheeses if you like, but I find this to be an unnecessary chore when there are so many delicious raw goat cheeses available on the market, which digest beautifully.

If it's a hearty meal of *starches* you crave, build a meal around any whole-grain, sprouted-grain product or baked root vegetable. These always go best with a big raw salad, which may include avocado, if desired, and can be followed by some high-quality whole-grain cookies! You will feel very nurtured and cozy after such a meal!

When you want to enjoy *fatty* flavors, you have the creaminess of pure, organic cream and butter to choose from, as well as avocados and raw oils. You may also find raw nuts helpful, but be sure to combine all of these items properly.

A Few Tips on How to Keep the Pleasure Flowing

- Learn how to make a few high-vibration dishes and how to get what you want at restaurants, so you can enjoy all aspects of dining at home as well as out with your friends.

- Focus on what you can have, not what you will no longer be eating. (It was enough for me to know that I'd be able to enjoy great wine, creamy avocados, a whole range of sweet flavors, fine goat cheeses, and dark chocolate—and never have to count calories, fat, or carb content again!)

- Figure out which foods and flavors you most enjoy, and then adapt them to the Raw Food Life Force Energy principles.

CUSTOMIZE IT ALL UNTIL IT FITS

Everyone has likes, dislikes, allergies, health issues, and numerous family, budget, and lifestyle considerations. All you have to do is plug your own needs, work hours, tastes, doctor's orders, and any other unique lifestyle scenarios into this program and you will see that it can work for you and everyone you know!

It is often said that one diet cannot work for everyone. That's not quite true. There is only one ideal diet, and that is one that moves quickly through the body, delivering lots of Life Force Energy. The only necessary adjustments depend on an individual's food preferences and appropriate level of transition away from a mainstream diet to this one. For example, if you cannot tolerate goat cheese or even the slightest amount of dairy, simply omit it. If you are a diabetic, stick to low-sugar fruits such as grapefruits and berries instead of going hog-wild on dates and raw honey! A little common sense is all it takes to personalize this diet to perfection.

First, customize the program to your daily schedule. I do this with all of my clients. You need to know what you're going to eat and when. Preparation is a large part of succeeding at this. *Second*, plan according to your personal likes and dislikes. If you don't like avocados and you see them in recipes or listed as an ideal food, you don't have to eat them. Choose another healthy option. If you're a strict vegetarian, ignore the fish and egg options. If you're allergic to nuts or seeds, just work around them. Nothing is mandatory except that you follow the basic principles. Eat what you want within the guidelines. It is also wise to eliminate foods that you know trigger bingeing for you—perhaps bread products, sugars (even natural ones), or wine.

HARMONY AT HOME

As a wife and mother myself, I can tell you that integrating this way of eating into the home is not as difficult as you might think. There is a very easy, practical approach. The key is never to force anyone else to do as you do. As a family leader, all you can do is set an example. Instead of telling my children what to eat, I give them lots of options and information. Don't underestimate your children's or your partner's ability to learn from observing you quietly making choices that transform your appearance and attitude. Such transformations are major draws and do not go unnoticed.

In order for the high-vibration raw living to work in the long term, it must create harmony, not division, in your home. Do whatever it takes to keep it fun, practical, and especially nonthreatening to your family without compromising your own dedication to eating for Life Force Energy. One of the best ways to do this is to make the best foods highly appealing, abundant, and readily available in the kitchen. If you want to nurture greater physical health and emotional balance in your children and/or spouse, this is a great place to start!

LIFE FORCE ENERGY CHILDREN

There is every reason to expose your children to Life Force Energy–rich foods and not a single reason not to. Today, more than ever, we need to make sure that our children understand how food can either heal or damage them. Children are bright and far more adaptable than we sometimes realize. I send my kids to school with fresh brown-bag lunches every day, full of their favorite healthy foods. My six-year-old daughter, Alexandra, would like to share her list of favorite foods with the kids in your family. She promises they will enjoy them!

Alexandra's List

Dried strawberries

"Just" brand dried persimmon

Larabars (particularly the apple and chocolate flavors)

Young Thai coconuts

The Raw Bakery's cocoa brownies

Organic Gourmet cookies

Alta Dena raw cheddar-style goat cheese grated on salad with beets, balsamic vinegar, and Stevia

Spelt or whole-wheat pancakes

Barbara's brown rice krispy cereal with agave nectar or raw honey and almond milk

All of the elixirs in the recipe section

Fresh coconut water

Raw almond butter and raw honey sandwiches on sprouted-grain bread

LāLoo's goat's milk ice cream

Organic eggs scrambled with raw Alta Dena goat cheese

Sprouted-grain cinnamon raisin bagels (by Alverado St. Bakery) with raw
honey

Bananas topped with pure maple syrup and 100 percent pure cocoa powder

Pink winter grapefruit wedges

"Pizza" made with sprouted-grain tortillas

Age of Aquarius Mac 'n' Cheese (see recipe, page 205)

Kamut pasta with sea salt and organic butter

Goat cheese sandwiches on sprouted-grain bread with Dijon mustard,
lettuce, and tomatoes

Avocado sandwiches on sprouted-grain bread with Dijon mustard, lettuce, tomatoes, and alfalfa sprouts

100 percent pure fruit spread (particularly the St. Dalfour brand) and organic butter on sprouted-grain bread

Carrot sticks dipped in pure maple syrup

Alexandra also asked me to share the following thoughts with you and your kids:

- "Mommy, tell them it tastes really good!"

- "Get lots of sunshine—it feels nice and warm. The flowers smell so good!"

- "If you want to be really sneaky, when your daddy's asleep in the morning and
he's left his chocolate by his bedside, you can sneak a piece of chocolate and
say, 'Daddy, the chocolate is in my mouth!'"

Keep in mind that every mother (and father) is a healer. Every time you
prepare a meal for your family members, you have the power to help heal their
physical, emotional, and psychological imbalances. Everything that you do as a
parent is meaningful—whether you are encouraging family walks instead of

watching television, teaching your teenagers how to look great and slim down in constructive, empowering ways, taking the time to educate yourself about childhood illnesses and their natural remedies, or going out of your way to get the highest-quality produce and natural bathroom products.

Children and teenagers have impressionable minds that are constantly bombarded with misguided messages from the media and their peers. Proper parenting in today's world means bringing children back to their natural state of health, happiness, and harmony. I have worked with enough young people to know that they are hungry for knowledge that will help keep them healthy and strong mentally, physically, and emotionally. As nurturers, we must share all that we know with them in a gentle, approachable way. The best way to do this is to be a living example to them.

PRACTICAL APPLICATION 10: TRANSITION GRADUALLY FROM YOUR OLD WAYS TO HIGH-VIBRATION RAW LIVING

Transition is important in all aspects of life, not just diet. Transition enables us to try something new, develop trust in the process, and then go deeper. Instead of shocking your system with an all-or-nothing approach, move gradually toward your goal and note your experiences along the way. Continue only as long as it feels good.

What does it really mean to transition in this context? The goal is to trigger cleansing with the most minimal amount of dietary change necessary to see results. Transitioning in this way ensures that the eliminative organs can keep up with the whole cleansing process by steadily moving the wastes out. If we draw up much more waste matter than our bodies can eliminate at any given time, our bodies will become congested and end up reabsorbing the waste in the bloodstream.

But keep in mind that, even if you transition gently, the cleansing process is more cyclical than linear. As you progress, you will likely see and feel positive results 95 percent of the time, but about 5 percent of the time you may experience temporary cleansing responses—such as headaches, nasal congestion, breakouts, and so on—and perhaps not feel or look your best. For example, you might feel better than ever in a month and then have a minor setback a week later. That is actually what you want to happen, as it will indicate that your body is drawing up more poison to be eliminated! Don't let the momentary discomfort distract you from realizing just how far you've come.

Also keep in mind that, as you become "cleaner," you become more in tune with your body, so you may notice a small imperfection that you would never have noticed before, when you had a lot more problems with your body. Try to keep it all in perspective. There is no immediate need to become "vegan" or "raw" or even "vegetarian" to start this healing process. Just remember that the healing process begins the moment you stop consuming unfit foods and begin embracing the dietary and environmental principles in this book.

Trans means "cross," and in this case we are transitioning or "crossing over" to another state of being. On the one side of transition is where you are now—at some degree of physical and energetic imbalance. On the other side is a state of perfect balance and vitality. Just as there are an infinite number of points between each integer in mathematics, there are an infinite number of points between imbalance and perfect balance, so find your starting point and focus on progress, not absolute perfection. Progress is all that matters, because with every step you take, you will experience new levels of well-being that you probably didn't even know were possible!

TRANSITION TIP: LEARN THE BEST WAYS TO CONSUME THE DENSER QUICK-EXIT FOODS

One of the best parts about this diet program is the delicious, richly satisfying food you will be enjoying. To ensure that you make consistent progress, here are some key tips on how best to eat the denser foods in this diet, such as the grains, nuts, dried fruits, and fleshes.

Grains

First of all, consume only high-quality grains—that is, whole (preferably sprouted) grains. The highest-quality, quick-exit grains are millet and quinoa. Spelt and kamut are also very good choices. They move through the digestive system even more quickly than whole wheat, and people who are allergic to wheat can often enjoy these grains. Eden Foods and VitaSpelt make wonderful pastas using these grains instead of wheat.

The key to grains is not to overeat them, but many people find it difficult to consume them in moderate amounts, and some women simply cannot lose weight while eating them. So, if your weight loss efforts have stalled, try nixing grains and see what happens. This grain problem usually goes hand in hand with the fruit problem, which is often indicative of *Candida* (or too much yeast in the system), so you'll want to tailor your detox diet accordingly. Yeast is a fungus that thrives in the presence of starches, fruits, and alcohol (to help combat fungus, try the Garden of Eden brand Fungal Defense and the OregaMax brand oil of oregano supplements). Once your system becomes clean enough (you'll know this has happened when you feel clear-headed, lose any excess weight, and experience excellent bowel elimination), you'll most likely be able to enjoy fresh fruits and some high-quality starches and wine again as a regular part of your diet. Do take your personal needs into account. We are all coming to this with very different life experiences and health histories.

If you have no problem with grains, enjoy them with lots of raw vegetables and, of course, never any nuts, fruit, dried fruit, or flesh, per our food-combining laws.

Nuts

Most people who are transitioning away from a mainstream diet can eat a fair helping of raw nuts (remember they are to be eaten raw only) without losing ground. I recommend that the maximum portion size for nuts be about four ounces, but you should adjust it according to how your body responds. While I can offer basic guidelines that work for almost everyone, there will always be that small percentage of people (usually women over forty) who simply do not get rapid results if they incorporate nuts. If you love nuts, for best results, enjoy them for lunch or dinner with unlimited raw vegetables. They combine beautifully with all dried fruits and with chocolate, bananas, and coconuts. The "raw treats" on the market today are snack foods such as chips, crackers, brownies, pies, and cakes that are made from all raw ingredients, which usually consist of some combination of raw nuts and dried fruits.

Dried Fruit

How much you can indulge in this dense sweet really comes down to the individual. I can eat fifteen dates in a sitting and not put on an ounce, while someone who is more sensitive to fruit sugars (typically because they have too much yeast in their system) should probably eat only about three to five dates. But it mainly depends on how much dense food you consume during the day. You cannot expect to feel "light" if you are eating grain for lunch, nuts and/or dried fruit as a snack, and more grain, nuts, or flesh for dinner. It's just too much density. (Note: dried fruits, young coconuts, and bananas go with avocados, but nuts do not mix with avocados.)

Avocados

Because they are much less dense than nuts, avocados are always the better choice to round out a meal. Forget about their fat content. Avocados are a highly quick-exit food and may be enjoyed fairly liberally. Use them to add creaminess to raw vegetable–based soups, to "beef" up a sandwich for lunch, to make a salad more satisfying, or to make delicious desserts and snacks such as raw chocolate pudding or guacamole. They combine beautifully with every vegetable and with all grains and cooked starch root vegetables. For a lovely, hearty supper, enjoy them over a salad with baked sweet potatoes!

PORTION SIZES

While measuring portion sizes is not critical, overeating is not helpful either. Use your intuition—you know how much is too much. For example, while you don't have to count out a specific number of nuts, don't sit down and eat a pound of cashews and think you're eating a cleansing meal! Here's a general guideline on how to approach portion sizes for the foods recommended in the Raw Food Life Force Energy diet:

Be as Generous as You Like

All raw vegetables

Fresh raw vegetable juices

Cooked non/low-starch vegetables

Young coconuts (don't confuse them with the "mature," hairy, brown coconuts; young coconuts are cut out of their big green shell and have
a white hard husk. They can be found in many Asian grocery stores,
and must be kept refrigerated.)

Fresh fruit (if it's on an empty stomach and you do not have diabetes, or
Candida, or get bloated when you eat fruit)

Be Fairly Generous but Do Not Overeat

Fish (up to three-fourths pound)

Sweet potatoes (one to three, medium size, depending on appetite)

Cooked starchy vegetables such as butternut or acorn squash (one to two cups)

Raw goat cheese (up to six or eight ounces)

Raw dried fruits (four to six ounces)

Be Careful Not to Overeat

Raw nuts (no more than four ounces)

Cooked whole grains such as brown rice, wheat berries, whole-grain pasta (up to one cup for women, two cups for men, preferably following only a raw vegetable salad; use cooked vegetables to "beef" up the plate)

Cow milk cheese or pasteurized cheeses (no more than two ounces)

Cooked legumes such as lentils, beans, cooked corn, cooked peas (up to one cup)

IF YOU SLIP, GET BACK IN THE GAME!

It will happen at some point: you're going strong and having tons of success on the program, then a few meals get away from you, and then these few meals turn into a couple of weeks of backsliding. This is typical during the holiday season or on a vacation. Almost everyone I have worked with has experienced this and temporarily struggled to get motivated again. There are a couple of reasons for this: (1) After a week or so of eating unfit foods, your body becomes less sensitive to them and they seem normal to your diet again, making you think you won't be satisfied without them. (2) You become less sensitive vibrationally and forget how light and clean you feel inside and out when you eat correctly.

Once your body is clean, or at least cleaner, and you consume too many inharmonious, low-vibration foods, you are probably going to feel sluggish and depressed. The chemicals in the food and your frustration with yourself may make you edgy and moody, which will only perpetuate the poor eating cycle. But how do you jump back in the game? In my practice and personal experience, I have found the following approaches to work almost all the time. Figure out the one that speaks to you and let it empower you in moments of weakness!

- Get back to vegetable juicing no matter what and take in nothing but raw vegetable juice (preferably Green Juice in a Pinch, page 163) until lunch or dinner for two days, followed by raw salads and steamed veggies at mealtime. These two days will resensitize your body and palate to the pleasures of this diet, help you recommit to it, and relieve the pressure in your bowels, which contributes to the lethargy and agitation you may be feeling.

- Set a plan that you can stick with that doesn't take you further off track than you already are. Nix all processed foods and poor combinations. If you are very far off the program, then just go back to the basics and work your way back a little more every day. Remember that the practical applications in this book work very quickly, and over the course of just a couple of days your body will respond!

- Have some body work done. Massage, lymphatic drainage, a colonic, and some hearty activity such as hiking, swimming, skiing, surfing, and so on. This will activate your body's ability to move poisons out through the skin and lymphatic system, making you feel cleaner and more joyful, which will help release you from damaging habits.

- Look at the new routines you've developed around your bad habits. Are you staying up late every night, drinking more than usual, watching too much TV, working late hours, under unusual stress at work or at home? Look at what you are doing that is separating you from your joyful self and then change it to the best of your ability. When we slip, there's usually an underlying emotional pattern at work. Once you can identify and shine a light on it, it is easier to change.

A REVIEW OF ALL THE PRACTICAL APPLICATIONS

Practical Application 1: Consume high–Life Force Energy foods.

Practical Application 2: Eliminate the food wastes from your body via colonics, body brushing, probiotics, alkalinity, and sweating.

Practical Application 3: Pump Life Force Energy through the body with the Life Force Energy Power Breath.

Practical Application 4: Enliven your body.

Practical Application 5: Eat "quick-exit" foods in "quick-exit" combinations.

Practical Application 6: Practice eating "light to heavy."

Practical Application 7: Remove the environmental obstacles between you and your natural joy.

Practical Application 8: Notice how modern thinking and living leach your natural joy.

Practical Application 9: Link pleasure, customization, and convenience.

Practical Application 10: Transition gradually from your old ways to this new diet and high-vibration raw living.

PART II

REBUILDING YOUR BODY IN 21 DAYS

A SUPERCHARGED ACTION PLAN

It's important that you follow this plan for a full 21 days because this period of time will enable you to learn new habits and set new patterns. Feel free to repeat the 21-day program as often as you like, with or without breaks in between. The goal is to give you what you need to overcome your food addictions and destructive patterns that have been engrained in you over decades. Ultimately, I hope that you will be so pleased with the results and that you will adopt this daily regimen for life!

Given the fact that everyone has a unique schedule and food preferences, feel free to adjust the meals and order of meals as they suit you. Just be sure to have your vegetable juice and probiotic on an empty stomach and apply "light-to-heavy" eating as often as possible. Advanced followers may wish to leave out the grain or nonlive foods listed for the lunchtime meals, but this is completely optional and recommended only for truly advanced followers. Additionally, be sure to customize the program, according to Practical Application 9, if you have any dietary restrictions.

Serving sizes of these meals are up to you. As long as you do not overeat, you may enjoy the amount that leaves you well satisfied. If your overall daily intake is high in Life Force Energy–rich foods (fresh fruits and veggies) and low in cooked and starchy foods, you can't go wrong. People often ask me how much of the dark chocolate they can eat. First, I recommend choosing a high-quality chocolate of 70 percent cocoa or more. My favorite brands are Green & Black and Dagoba. Try to limit it to fifty grams a day (which is a generous portion consisting of half of an entire large Green & Black bar).

A FEW STEPS BEFORE YOU START TO ENSURE A SMOOTH AND SUCCESSFUL TRANSITION

Prepare Your Kitchen

Clear out your cabinets, refrigerator, and freezer of the unfit foods of your past.

Shop for Staples

Pick up the basic nonperishable and semiperishable items that you will use daily. Doing this ahead of time will ensure that you have on hand many of the ingredients for the recipes you'll want to prepare at home. It will also keep your shopping list as short as possible!

Lemons and/or limes
Balsamic vinegar
Cold-pressed olive oil
Celtic sea salt
Fresh peppercorns in a pepper mill
Fresh garlic
Fresh ginger
Alta Dena raw cheddar-style goat cheese

Organic carrots

Organic Dijon-style mustard (I like the Westbrae Natural brand best)

Organic butter

Nama Shoyu (raw soy sauce)

Pure maple syrup and/or agave nectar

Raw honey (the "Really Raw" brand is my favorite)

Stevia (NuNaturals brand)

Green & Black or Dagoba 70 percent + Dark Chocolate

Revise the Way You Shop

- Check labels for unfit ingredients before buying packaged foods.

- Make every effort to shop at the highest-quality organic markets.

- Take advantage of grocery delivery services to make getting your fresh ingredients as easy as possible.

- If you like dried fruits, use only the unsulfured, unsweetened variety.

21 DAYS OF QUICK-EXIT LUNCHES, DINNERS, SNACKS, AND DESSERTS

One of the best things about this way of eating is how much you can mix and match recipes to suit your personal tastes, keep your palate happy, and stay within your budget. Once you get the hang of the combinations that make for a quick-exit meal, you will be able to mix and match easily. To take the guess work out of it completely, the following pages have 21 lunch and dinner suggestions followed by desserts that can be enjoyed within each category of food. *Just remember that like categories combine with like categories and everything in the neutral category. It's that easy.*

Since we all have varying appetites, I urge you to refer to the following meal suggestions merely as a guide. You may find some of the combinations I list in the program to be too filling, in which case you may just pick one of the two dishes offered—for example, have the salad and leave out the soup or the cooked dish. Or you may want every course *and* seconds. The goal is to ensure that you are satisfied and inspired over the long term, so take or leave whichever offerings suit you. Once you've decided what you would like to eat, check the information on desserts to know which desserts you could pair with each lunch and dinner option. Note that while there are some light, cooked foods that you may incorporate in the middle of the day, most of the cooked suggestions are for dinnertime.

LUNCHES

1. Salad Gone Nuts (page 181) and Nut-Butter and Jelly Sandwiches (page 197)

2. The Daily Avocado Classic (page 180) and Pumpkin Pie in a Bowl (page 166)

3. Salad Sandwich (page 200) and Cleansing Corn Chowder (page 168)

4. Avocado Wrap (page 199) and Raw Cream of Tomato Soup (page 167)

5. Salad Gone Nuts (page 181) with Raw Open-Faced Sandwiches (page 197)

6. Portobello-Marinara Grandwich (page 198) and fresh greens with Quick Balsamic Dressing (page 174)

7. Grain-free Asian Kombu Noodle Soup (page 170) with Ak-Mak brand crackers and greens with Sesame Gingersnap Dressing (page 175)

8. Pineapple's Just Peachy Summer Soup (page 171) followed five to ten minutes later (to give the fruit soup a head start)* by the Raw Open-Faced Sandwiches (page 197)

9. Don't Lose Your Tacos (page 189) with raw corn on the cob and/or baked sweet potato

10. Sweet Potato Beet Pasta with Pesto and Diced Tomatoes (page 191)

11. Quickest Spaghetti (page 195) with any raw crackers

12. Bagels and "Green" Cheese (page 218) with Summer Salad, Poolside (page 183) and a dollop of Salsa Mole (page 220)

13. Nut-Butter and Jelly Sandwiches (page 197) and your favorite raw vegetables

14. Raw Open-Faced Sandwiches (page 197) and Turkish Three-Pepper Tomato Salad (page 185)

15. Powerful Beet-Parsley Cleansing Salad (page 185) with the Best Thing Since Sliced Bread (page 218)

16. Turkish Three-Pepper Tomato Salad (page 185) and Raw Cream of Tomato (page 167)

---

*Blended fruit moves through the stomach faster than whole fruit since it is broken down by the blender.

17. Suddenly St. Tropez (page 179) and steamed vegetables

18. Sun-Dried Summer Slimmer (page 182) and Raw Tomato Herb Potage with Shredded Raw Goat Cheese (page 169)

19. Daily Avocado Classic (page 180) and a baked sweet potato

20. Fresh fruit salad followed by Milk that Shakes & Shapes (page 223) or Chocolate Mousse (page 223)

21. An entrée size portion of mixed greens and other raw vegetables of your choice topped with plenty of Creamy Herb Live Yogurt Dressing (page 177) and unlimited steamed vegetables

DINNERS

You may have any of the above-mentioned lunches for dinner as well, but if you prefer heavier, cooked foods like the ones below, keep in mind that it's best to have them at the end of the day. I recommend always accompanying a cooked meal with some raw vegetables. This can be in the form of anything from some very simple greens or cut up vegetables and carrot sticks, to one of the raw salad recipes in this book. Then, if you have a sweet tooth, you can check the upcoming list of desserts to find which ones to pair with these dinner options.

1. Sushi to Impress (page 188) and a simple green salad with Sesame Gingersnap Dressing (page 175)

2. Don't Lose Your Cheesy Tacos (page 190) and Raw Tomato Herb Potage with Shredded Raw Goat Cheese (page 169)

3. Portobello Melts (page 198) and Sun-Dried Summer Slimmer (page 182)

4. Portobello Steaks and Burgers (page 204) and simple greens with Quick Balsamic Dressing (page 174)

5. Portobello-Marinara Grandwich (page 198) and Sandwich Salad (page 186)

6. Parsnip-Carrot-Beet Bake (page 202) and sweet potatoes with greens and sliced avocado topped with Quick Balsamic Dressing (page 174)

7. Raw Teriyaki "Stir-Fry" (page 194)

8. Sweet Butternut Heaven (page 206) and Mega-Veggie Platter (page 206)

9. Mega-Veggie Platter (page 206) with baked sweet potato and simple greens dressed with Quick Balsamic Dressing (page 174)

10. Red Beet Ravioli Stuffed with Tarragon Goat Cheese (page 192) and simple leafy green salad dressed with Quick Balsamic Dressing (page 174)

11. Kombu Melt (page 208) and Sweet Basil Tomato Towers (page 207)

12. No-Fry Stir-Fry (page 209)

13. Age of Aquarius Mac 'n' Cheese (page 205) and Summer Salad, Poolside (page 183)

14. Beet This Flounder! (page 211) and Turkish Three-Pepper Tomato Salad (page 185)

15. Simple Spiked Snapper (page 212) and Powerful Beet-Parsley Cleansing
    Salad (page 184)

16. Has-to-Be Halibut (page 212) with Sweet Chili-Lime Dressing (page 174)

17. Herb-Encrusted Swordfish (page 213) and Turkish Three-Pepper Tomato
    Salad (page 185)

18. The Best Thing Since Sliced Bread (page 218) and sweet potatoes and
    simple greens dressed with Quick Balsamic (page 174)

19. Daily Avocado Classic (page 180) with Parsnip-Carrot-Beet Bake (page 202)

20. Powerful Beet-Parsley Cleansing Salad (page 184) and Pumpkin Pie in a
    Bowl (page 166)

21. Suddenly St. Tropez (page 179) and Raw Tomato Herb Potage with
    Shredded Raw Goat Cheese (page 169)

DESSERTS

The following dessert suggestions are for any meals in the "flesh" category:

Dark chocolate
Raw cheese

The following dessert suggestions are for any meals in the "starch" category:

Dark chocolate

Young coconut

Whole-grain cookies

The following dessert suggestions are for any meals in the "all raw, nut-based" category:

Dates or dried fruit

Dark chocolate

"Baked" Apples (page 226)

Raw Granola (page 219)

Lemon Meringue Mousse (page 225)

Chocolate Mousse (page 223)

Milk that Shakes & Shapes (page 223)

The following dessert suggestions are for any meals in the "all raw, avocado-based" category:

"Baked" Apples (page 226)

Lemon Meringue Mouse (page 225) Chocolate Mousse (page 223)

Milk That Shakes & Shapes (page 223)

SNACKS

Some people need to eat constantly and others can go long stretches between meals effortlessly. To the latter group, I say, don't start a habit of snacking if you don't have one already. Snacking makes the digestive system work around the clock, which will make you feel fatigued and slow the whole cleansing/healing process. For those of you who want, or need, food between meals, reach for the quickest-exit foods—namely, fresh fruits and vegetables. The goal is to select mini-meals that require minimal digestive effort.

Raw vegetables are the most ideal snack because they are light and will not create fermentation if you eat them too soon after lunch. Fresh fruits are a good snack if you wait a full three hours after a properly combined lunch. Nuts/seeds/dried fruits are okay if you wait a full three hours after a properly combined, nut-free lunch and a full three hours before a nut-free dinner. For example, if you enjoy the Salad Gone Nuts for lunch, you may enjoy anything made from nuts/seeds/dried fruits anytime as dessert or a snack without waiting any specific amount of time.

I recommend snacking from the same category of food as your lunch to eliminate the issue of waiting, which is why in the 21-day program I have mostly incorporated snacks that don't require a waiting period. What many of my clients like to do is split their lunch up into two parts. For example, if they had an avocado sandwich and salad at midday, they might have more of that sandwich or another avocado sandwich (possibly with any leftover salad or vegetables) midafternoon. Since whole-grain cookies combine with the grain-bread sandwiches, they could also have some whole-grain cookies later on without having to worry about what the midday lunch has left in the stomach. The other way to avoid waiting is to eat a neutral meal before your snack. For example, if you just eat a large raw vegetable salad for lunch, which is completely neutral, you can enjoy a snack from any category at snack time. If you prefer to have a late-day snack, you could select one from the same food group as your dinner. For example, if you knew you were having fish and vegetables for dinner at 7 P.M. but you wanted a snack at 5 or 6 P.M., you could enjoy some raw goat cheese and vegetables because they combine perfectly with fish.

DRINKS

Try to avoid drinking a lot with meals, as liquid will dilute your digestive power. In between meals, enjoy clean water, fresh fruit and vegetable juice, herbal teas, the Kombucha Digestif (page 164), or any of the other elixirs in the recipe section. But note that the vegetable elixirs should be enjoyed on an empty stomach for maximum benefit and digestibility.

Although wine, like chocolate, is compatible with this diet program, I do not believe that these substances offer physiological benefits, despite what some studies and news stories say. But when consumed in moderation, these substances don't interfere with the cleansing process, and they can help make the whole process more fun, approachable, sociable, and pleasing to the senses—which is important!

THE LIFE FORCE ENERGY BODY TEST

Take the following test to see how you score and then get started with Day 1!

How filled with Life Force Energy are you today? Take this test and find out! Please keep in mind that the point of this test is not to get the highest possible score. Getting a low score means only that you will undergo a radical transformation over the next 21 days, and that you should be very excited about! Whatever your score, you'll be able to grow exponentially more youthful, attractive, and emotionally balanced as you go deeper with this program.

1. (a) I am relaxed and happy most of the time.
   (b) I manage my emotions but I'd prefer to be more centered.
   (c) I am generally quite nervous and/or edgy.

2. (a) I am doing positive things with my time and/or have a job that allows me to express my natural talents and creativity.
   (b) I don't feel like I've found my calling but I do have a lot of hobbies.

(c) I really don't enjoy my job, but it's a living for me right now and may always be.

3. Please finish the following sentence: I like what I see in the mirror . . .
   (a) a lot.
   (b) somewhat.
   (c) not at all.

4. (a) I see other people as my equal in all ways and worthy of the very best in life.
   (b) Sometimes I feel generous toward people, and other times—usually when I'm wound up with my own issues—I don't treat them as well as I could.
   (c) I think some people are more deserving of good things than others.

5. (a) I am the kind of person who counts my blessings.
   (b) I'm working so hard to keep things going in my life that I often forget to pause and be grateful for what I've done and what I have. I'd love to have a moment to reflect on the good things in my life, but I always have something else to do.
   (c) I am often critical of my life and what I lack.

6. How true is the following statement for you? I am very happy with my weight.
   (a) Completely
   (b) Somewhat
   (c) Not at all

7. (a) I have learned how to enjoy the simple pleasure of breathing deeply.

    (b) Sometimes I remember to focus on breathing deeply, but often I forget.

    (c) I don't really pay attention to my breathing.

8. (a) I spend a lot of time out in nature.

    (b) Even though I don't spend a lot of time in nature, I go outside for walks, sleep with my windows open, and take in sun whenever I can during safe hours.

    (c) I'm rarely in a natural environment or exposed to natural elements.

9. Please finish the following sentence: If it is true that like attracts like, I would be attracting . . .

    (a) the best life has to offer.

    (b) mediocre opportunities and relationships.

    (c) a pretty miserable lot.

10. Please finish the following sentence: I enjoy the food I usually eat . . .

    (a) a lot.

    (b) somewhat.

    (c) not at all. I feel very deprived.

11. How often do you eat when you're not hungry and/or before you're sure that your last meal has passed through your stomach?

    (a) Never

    (b) Somewhat

    (c) Practically always

12. (a) I feel the tingle of Life Force Energy flowing through me more and more.

    (b) I am intuitively aware of my energy body and the Life Force Energy in and around me, but I don't feel it strongly yet.

    (c) I haven't ever felt the tingle of Life Force Energy flowing through me and, until now, I didn't even know it existed.

13. (a) I eat harmoniously vibrating foods almost all the time.

    (b) I eat some harmoniously vibrating foods, but mainly I eat what's available.

    (c) I eat a pretty incoherent range of foods, now that I think about it.

14. (a) I practice yoga, dance, or some form of deep breathing exercise daily.

    (b) I am doing some form of deep breathing exercise a couple of times a week.

    (c) I haven't done any of these types of exercise in years, if ever.

15. (a) I schedule some form of body work (such as massage, self-massage, rolfing, etc.) as often as possible, and I dry brush my body at least several times a week.

    (b) I need to start incorporating massage and body brushing into my routine.

16. (a) I believe that I can be radiant and spend my time doing things I love, and that my life will get consistently more enjoyable as the years go by.

(b) While I'm not there yet, I am confident that I am going to have a breakthrough and experience all the great things that this program promises in the coming weeks and months.

(c) I'm not entirely convinced that life can be great or that I'll ever look or feel radiant.

17. (a) I'm learning to express myself more, listen to my intuition, and pursue my dreams.

(b) If I remember my dreams and tune into my inner voice, I think I'll be able to improve my life.

(c) I feel pretty rigid and find it hard to express myself, but I'm going to try to get better at it.

Score yourself: Add up all your (a)'s, (b)'s and (c)'s. Give yourself 3 points for every (a), 2 points for every (b), and 1 point for every (c) for a total of 51 possible points.

IF YOU'VE SCORED 46 TO 51 POINTS: I don't even need to ask how you're vibing! Well done. You are one radiant energy body. The world needs your light, so keep it up and spread the message! For you, I recommend more of the same with more acute attention to eliminating toxins through the skin and colon, enlivening the body through yoga, breath, dance, and massage, and summoning ever greater harmony and higher vibration energy as you are ready. Yours is, and will continue to be, a lifetime of bliss!

IF YOU'VE SCORED 37 TO 45 POINTS: You are not down-and-out, but you're not feeling nearly as good as you could. If you focus on the practical applications in this book, you will soon experience far superior states of physical beauty and emotional well-being. I recommend close adherence to the guidelines of transition, focusing on your food combinations, body-enlivening techniques, and really becoming aware of your energy body. You're on your way to a lifetime of bliss . . .

IF YOU'VE SCORED 17 TO 37 POINTS: If I could climb into your body, take it over, restore it to its natural vibration, and hand it back to you, I would. But I can't, so you are going to have to do it with me as your guide. I will be with you every step of the way and cheering you on at every goal line! Don't be afraid to dream. I'm here to help you make your dreams come true! But remember to transition with care—this is not a race. If you can focus on only two practical applications right now, I would suggest they be quick-exit combinations and enlivening the body through breath work, yoga, and dance.

21 DAYS OF THE RAW FOOD LIFE FORCE ENERGY PROGRAM

DAY 1

UPON RISING: Dry brush thoroughly using your natural-bristle body brush, then devote some time to a body-enlivening practice of your choice (formal or informal yoga sequences, Tai Chi, simple stretching, or dance, as discussed on pages (53–55).*

PRE-BREAKFAST: Vegetable juice should be the first thing you ingest today, but you do not need to drink it right away. If you prefer, drink it later in the morning or throughout the morning, as long as it's on an empty stomach. Enjoy a minimum of eight to sixteen ounces of Life Force Power-ade (page 158) or The Great Eliminator (page 158).

---

*You can spend as little or as much time on your body-enlivening techniques as you like. Remember, it is not about duration, but about committing to these activities on a regular basis and deriving enjoyment from them.

BEFORE LEAVING HOME: Use the Life Force Power Breath (see page 51) for at least one full minute (try it in the shower). Take the time to move your bowels. For a more efficient elimination, keep your feet elevated four to ten inches off the floor on a stool or an upside-down wastebasket. *Do this every morning*, whether you feel you're ready to go or not, so that it will set your intestinal clock.*

BREAKFAST: Enjoy any of the elixirs and/or fresh fruit as desired, stopping thirty minutes before your lunchtime meal.

LUNCH: Choose the most desirable meal from pages 100–102 or a well-combined meal of your own. Have as much or as little as you need. While you're eating lunch, consider your emotional ties to food. Don't be self-critical, just let the ideas flow and make a note of them. You might try the Daily Avocado Classic (page 180) and Pumpkin Pie in a Bowl (page 166). Since the soup recipe makes more than four cups, have more of it as a snack with some salad, bananas, or dates, if desired, whenever you like.

PRE-DINNER (OPTIONAL): 1 pound of raw carrots or other desired raw vegetable(s) with your favorite alkalinizing dipping sauce.

DINNER: Choose the most desirable dinner/dessert combination from pages 102–4 or a well-combined meal of your own. You might try the Has-to-Be Halibut (page 212) with the Sweet Chili-Lime Dressing (page 174) and have some of the Green & Black 70 percent chocolate for dessert.

---

*To avoid unnecessary repetition, this is the only time I will instruct you to eliminate before leaving home, but be sure to do so every day at roughly the same time.

BEFORE RETIRING: Take some time to thoroughly unwind. Soak in a hot bath (try adding in a container of Epsom salts, which are great for eliminating toxins). At some point, whether you are doing chores, watching TV, reading, or just spending time with your family, focus on breathing in fresh air for one full minute using the Life Force Power Breath.

HOMEWORK: Write down, in as much detail as possible, what your current physical, mental, and spiritual states are. How do you feel about them?

On a scale from 1 to 10 (10 being the highest), how would you rate your level of Life Force Energy today?

NOTES:

DAY 2

UPON RISING: Dry brush thoroughly using your natural-bristle body brush, then devote some time to a body-enlivening practice of your choice.

PRE-BREAKFAST: Enjoy a minimum of eight to sixteen ounces of either Life Force Power-ade (page 158) or The Great Eliminator (page 158) on an empty stomach.

BEFORE LEAVING HOME: Use the Life Force Power Breath (page 51) for at least one full minute (try it while you decide what to wear—you'll probably put together something more inspired!).

BREAKFAST: Enjoy any of the elixirs in the recipe section and/or fresh fruit as desired, stopping thirty minutes before your lunchtime meal.

LUNCH: Choose the most desirable meal from pages 100–102 or a well combined meal of your own. Have as much or as little as you need. While you're eating lunch, be mindful of the purpose of food and how overeating drains you of the energy that you need throughout the day. You might try the Salad Gone Nuts (page 181) and the Nut-Butter and Jelly Sandwiches (page 197). As with all the lunches, you may enjoy it all at once or, if you prefer, save some of it as a snack for later.

DINNER: Choose the most desirable dinner/dessert combination from pages 102–4 or a well-combined meal of your own. You might try the Portobello Steaks and Burgers (page 204) and a mixed greens salad dressed with Quick Balsamic (page 174) and then enjoy the Kollar or Organic Gourmet whole-grain cookies or dark chocolate for a dessert.

BEFORE RETIRING: Take some time to thoroughly unwind. Tonight, try massaging your feet and legs with natural oils. At some point, whether you are doing chores, watching TV, reading, or just spending time with your family, focus on breathing fresh air for one full minute using the Life Force Power Breath.

HOMEWORK: Write down your long-term goal for your body and how you are going to achieve it. Note how you feel in your body now, then visualize yourself in the body you want and imagine how you will feel in it.

On a scale of 1 to 10, how would you rate your level of Life Force Energy today?

NOTES:

DAY 3

UPON RISING: Dry brush thoroughly using your natural-bristle body brush, then devote some time to a body-enlivening activity of your choice. Employ a gravity-method enema (or colonic) now or at some convenient time during the day when your stomach is empty.

PRE-BREAKFAST: Enjoy a minimum of eight to sixteen ounces of either Life Force Power-ade (page 158) or The Great Eliminator (page 158) on an empty stomach.

BEFORE LEAVING HOME: Use the Life Force Power Breath for at least one full minute (try it while watching the morning news).

BREAKFAST: Enjoy any of the elixirs in the recipe section and/or fresh fruit as desired, stopping thirty minutes before your lunchtime meal.

LUNCH: Choose the most desirable meal from pages 100–102 or a well-combined meal of your own. Have as much or as little as you need. While you're eating lunch, consider how the food you are eating is enabling healing to take place in your body. You might try the Avocado Wrap (page 199) and Raw Cream of Tomato Soup (page 167) and have some Ak-Mak crackers as a dessert.

DINNER: Choose the most desirable dinner/dessert combination from pages 102–4. You might try the Raw Teriyaki "Stir-Fry" (page 194) followed by a brownie from The Raw Bakery and/or a cup of raw chocolate ice cream for dessert.

BEFORE RETIRING: Take some time to thoroughly unwind. Tonight, try massaging your hands and arms with natural oils. Use a calming, pure essential oil such as lavender, lemon, lemongrass, orange, or ylang ylang (do not use stimulating oils close to bedtime). Place three drops of your favorite scent in the middle of one palm. Rub your palms vigorously together and then bring your palms to your nose and breathe it in. It's very soothing and will help put you to sleep when you're ready. At some point, be sure to practice the Life Force Power Breath for two full, conscious minutes.

HOMEWORK: Reflect on your long-term goal, which you wrote down yesterday, and write down the things you do that distract you from your goal. Then write down who or what is responsible for distracting you from that goal. Then visualize removing all possible distractions and achieving your long term goal.

On a scale of 1 to 10, how would you rate your level of Life Force Energy today?

NOTES:

DAY 4

UPON RISING: Dry brush thoroughly using your natural-bristle body brush, then devote some time to a body-enlivening practice of your choice.

PRE-BREAKFAST: Enjoy a minimum of eight to sixteen ounces of Life Force Power-ade or The Great Eliminator on an empty stomach.

BEFORE LEAVING HOME: Use the Life Force Power Breath for at least one full minute (try it while putting on your makeup or skin cream).

BREAKFAST: Enjoy any of the elixirs in the recipe section and/or fresh fruit as desired, stopping thirty minutes before your lunchtime meal.

LUNCH: Choose the most desirable option from pages 100–102 or a well-combined meal of your own. Have as much or as little as you need. While you're eating lunch, imagine the food raising your vibrations and focus on the sensation of your energy body all around you. You might try the Portobello-Marinara Grandwich (page 198) and fresh greens dressed with Quick Balsamic Dressing (page 174), then after waiting three full hours enjoy a couple of bananas or some fresh carrot juice.

DINNER: Choose the most desirable dinner/dessert combination from pages 102–4 or a well-combined meal of your own. You might try the Herb-Encrusted Swordfish (page 213) and the Turkish Three-Pepper Tomato Salad (page 185) and have some dark chocolate and/or a bit of raw goat cheese for dessert.

BEFORE RETIRING: Take some time to thoroughly unwind. Tonight, try massaging your face when you apply your moisturizer. Finish by massaging your ears and scalp and feel the tension release. At some point, be sure to practice the Life Force Power Breath for two full, conscious minutes.

HOMEWORK: Write down what you would do with your life if no one could criticize or praise you. How would you spend your time? Would you create something? If so, what? Would your life be very different? What does this tell you about how much power you give to other people? Just take a moment to explore this idea. You don't need to have all the answers. Being honest with yourself is the most important part of this exercise. On a scale of 1 to 10, how would you rate your level of Life Force Energy today?

NOTES:

DAY 5

UPON RISING: Dry brush thoroughly using your natural-bristle body brush, then devote some time to a body-enlivening practice of your choice.

PRE-BREAKFAST: Enjoy a minimum of eight to sixteen ounces of Life Force Power-ade or The Great Eliminator on an empty stomach.

BEFORE LEAVING HOME: Use the Life Force Power Breath for at least one full minute (try it while emptying the dishes from the dishwasher or doing some other household chore).

BREAKFAST: Enjoy any of the elixirs in the recipe section and/or fresh fruit as desired, stopping thirty minutes before your lunchtime meal.

LUNCH: Choose the most desirable meal from pages 100–102 or a well-combined meal of your own. Have as much or as little as you need. While you're eating lunch, think about the environment you're eating in. Is it conducive to oxygenating your body? Are you physically comfortable? You might try the Sweet Potato Beet Pasta with Pesto and Diced Tomatoes (page 191) and have a Raw Bakery chocolate brownie and a cup of herbal tea sweetened with Stevia for a dessert.

DINNER: Choose the most desirable dinner/dessert combination from pages 102–4 or a well-combined meal of your own. You might try the Daily Avocado Classic (page 180) with the Parsnip-Carrot-Beet Bake (page 202) and enjoy an Organic Gourmet chocolate chip cookie and a cup of herbal tea with stevia for dessert.

BEFORE RETIRING: Take some time to thoroughly unwind. If the weather permits, go for a long walk, feel your body relax and feel more connected to the outdoors with every stride. At some point, be sure to practice the Life Force Power Breath for three full, conscious minutes.

HOMEWORK: Think about the body-enlivening activities you've practiced and how they make you feel. Which ones might you like to try in the coming days?

On a scale of 1 to 10, how would you rate your level of Life Force Energy today?

NOTES:

DAY 6

UPON RISING: Dry brush thoroughly using your natural-bristle body brush, then devote some time to a body-enlivening practice of your choice.

PRE-BREAKFAST: Enjoy a minimum of eight to sixteen ounces of Life Force Power-ade or The Great Eliminator on an empty stomach.

BEFORE LEAVING HOME: Use the Life Force Power Breath for at least two full minutes (try it while making your bed).

BREAKFAST: Enjoy any of the elixirs in the recipe section and/or fresh fruit as desired, stopping thirty minutes before your lunchtime meal.

LUNCH: Choose the most desirable option from pages 100–102 or a well-combined meal of your own. Have as much or as little as you need. While you're eating lunch, imagine the food you are eating moving seamlessly through your body, giving you nourishment without leaving any heaviness behind. You might try the Bagels and "Green" Cheese (page 218) with the Summer Salad, Poolside (page 183) and a dollop of Salsa Mole (page 220), and have whatever you don't finish anytime later as your snack.

DINNER: Choose the most desirable dinner/dessert combination from page 102 or a well-combined meal of your own. You might try the Simple Spiked Snapper (page 212) and Powerful Beet-Parsley Cleansing Salad (page 184) and have some dark chocolate and/or a few slices of the Alta Dena raw cheddar-style goat cheese for dessert.

BEFORE RETIRING: Take some time to thoroughly unwind. Tonight, take a break from the Life Force Power Breath and try some meditation—either guided with a CD or just sit with your legs crossed in a quiet, peaceful place where you won't be disturbed. For at least five minutes or so, quiet your mind while you exhale any staleness from the day and inhale calmly to pave the way for a restful night's sleep.

HOMEWORK: Which harmful foods are you most addicted to? Write down five alkalinizing and oxygenating foods that you can eat in their place (you can use the recipe list on page 153 for ideas). Think about how light and energized they make you feel!

On a scale of 1 to 10, how would you rate your level of Life Force Energy today?

NOTES:

DAY 7

UPON RISING: Dry brush thoroughly with a natural-bristle body brush, then devote some time to a body-enlivening activity of your choice.

PRE-BREAKFAST: Enjoy a minimum of eight to sixteen ounces of Life Force Powerade or The Great Eliminator on an empty stomach.

BEFORE LEAVING HOME: Use the Life Force Power Breath for at least two full minutes (try it while clipping or filing your nails).

BREAKFAST: Enjoy any of the elixirs in the recipe section and/or fresh fruit as desired, stopping thirty minutes before your lunchtime meal.

LUNCH: Choose the most desirable option from pages 100–102 or a well-combined meal of your own. Have as much or as little as you need. While you're eating lunch think about how far you have come in just one week! You might try the Powerful Beet-Parsley Cleansing Salad (page 185) with The Best Thing Since Sliced Bread (page 218) and enjoy a couple of bananas as a snack.

DINNER: Choose the most desirable dinner/dessert combination from pages 102–4 or a well-combined meal of your own. You might try the No-Fry Stir-Fry (page 209) with a cup of brown rice and organic butter. Enjoy a bag of Kollar cookies for a dessert—three small-medium-sized cookies come in each bag.

BEFORE RETIRING: Enjoy any evening activity of your choice—a massage, a hot bath, a walk, or meditation—that appeals to you. Be sure to take time to practice the Life Force Power Breath for three full, conscious minutes.

HOMEWORK: When are you going on your next trip? List five things you can do to follow this program while you're traveling. Consider how you will get your vegetable juice or use a powder supplement, how you will ensure getting fresh fruits and vegetables and well-combined meals in restaurants, hotels, airplanes. Envision yourself taking these steps so that you will be lean and vibrant throughout your trip! On a scale of 1 to 10, how would you rate your level of Life Force Energy today?

NOTES:

DAY 8

UPON RISING: Dry brush thoroughly with your natural-bristle body brush, then devote some time to a body-enlivening activity of your choice.

PRE-BREAKFAST: Enjoy a minimum of eight to sixteen ounces of Life Force Power-ade or The Great Eliminator on an empty stomach.

BEFORE LEAVING HOME: Use the Life Force Power Breath for at least two full minutes (try it while folding your laundry).

BREAKFAST: Enjoy any of the elixirs in the recipe section and/or fresh fruit as desired, stopping thirty minutes before your lunchtime meal.

LUNCH: Choose the most desirable option from pages 100–102 or a well-combined meal of your own. Have as much or as little as you need. While you're eating lunch, fully relax and savor each bite. You might try the Grain-free Asian Kombu Noodle Soup (page 170) or the Sensei Said Soba Noodle Soup (page 172) with Ak-Mak brand crackers, and greens with Sesame Gingersnap Dressing (page 175), then have whatever you don't finish any time later as a snack.

DINNER: Choose the most desirable dinner/dessert combination from pages 102–4 or a well-combined meal of your own. You might try the Beet this Flounder! (page 211) and the Turkish Three-Pepper Tomato Salad (page 185), and have some dark chocolate for dessert.

BEFORE RETIRING: Enjoy any evening activity of your choice—a massage, a hot bath, a walk, or meditation—that appeals to you. At some point, practice the Life Force Power Breath for four full, conscious minutes.

Take the Life Force Energy Test on page 109 again and see how your score has changed since you first took it. Write your score here:

HOMEWORK: Now that you've completed one full week of the program, make a laundry list of what's working and what's not working. Next to each thing that is working, write why it works for you. Next to each thing that isn't working, write down at least one way to make it work. For example, if you're not feeling satisfied by a certain meal or a certain type of meal, you might write: "Find a more satisfying lunchtime meal" or "Need to eat more of X to feel satisfied." On a scale of 1 to 10, how would you rate your level of Life Force Energy today?

NOTES:

DAY 9

UPON WAKING: Use the Life Force Power Breath for at least two full minutes.

UPON RISING: Dry brush thoroughly using your natural-bristle body brush, then devote some time to a body-enlivening activity of your choice. Employ a gravity-method enema (or colonic) now or at some convenient time during the day when your stomach is empty.

PRE-BREAKFAST: Enjoy a minimum of eight to sixteen ounces of Life Force Power-ade or The Great Eliminator on an empty stomach.

BREAKFAST: Enjoy any of the elixirs in the recipe section and/or fresh fruit as desired, stopping thirty minutes before your lunchtime meal.

LUNCH: Choose the most desirable option from pages 100–102 or a well-combined meal of your own. Have as much or as little as you need. While you're eating lunch, ask yourself if you are more aware of the reasons why you eat (or used to eat) unnatural, low-vibration foods and whether you're improving your eating patterns. You might try the Daily Avocado Classic (page 180) with a baked sweet potato, and then enjoy some raw vegetables later for a snack.)

DINNER: Choose the most desirable dinner/dessert combination from pages 102–4 or a well-combined meal of your own. You might try the Sushi to Impress (page 188) and a simple green salad with Sesame Gingersnap Dressing (page 175), then if there's still room for dessert, enjoy some custard or the raw chocolate ice cream.

BEFORE RETIRING: Enjoy any evening activity of your choice—a massage, a hot bath, a walk, or meditation—that appeals to you. At some point, practice the Life Force Power Breath for four full, conscious minutes.

HOMEWORK: Write down all the benefits you are witnessing and feeling within your body as you follow this program. Consider how much pleasure you are deriving from this way of eating. On a scale of 1 to 10, how would you rate your level of Life Force Energy today?

NOTES:

DAY 10

UPON RISING: Dry brush thoroughly with your natural-bristle body brush, then devote some time to a body-enlivening activity of your choice.

PRE-BREAKFAST: Enjoy a minimum of eight to sixteen ounces of Life Force Power-ade or The Great Eliminator on an empty stomach.

BEFORE LEAVING HOME: Use the Life Force Power Breath for at least two full minutes (try it while getting dressed).

BREAKFAST: Enjoy any of the elixirs in the recipe section and/or fresh fruit as desired, stopping thirty minutes before your lunchtime meal.

LUNCH: Choose the most desirable option from pages 100–102 or a well-combined meal of your own. Have as much or as little as you need. While you're eating lunch, reflect upon this concept: Waste = Weight. Consider how unfit foods remain in the body and weigh you down. Visualize your body lifting, releasing the old waste matter and creating a home for rapidly flowing Life Force Energy instead! You might try to fast this morning on just vegetable juice and then enjoy fresh fruit throughout the afternoon, followed by Milk That Shakes & Shapes (page 223) or Chocolate Mousse (page 223) as a snack.

DINNER: Choose the most desirable dinner/dessert combination from pages 102–4 or a well-combined meal of your own. You might try the Portobello Melts (page 203) and the Sun-Dried Summer Slimmer (page 182) and have some dark chocolate for a dessert.

BEFORE RETIRING: Enjoy any evening activity of your choice—a massage, a hot bath, a walk, or meditation—that appeals to you. Be sure to make time to practice the Life Force Power Breath for four full, conscious minutes.

HOMEWORK: Consider the messages we get from the media every day. Do you think they are for your benefit or for the benefit of big business? Can you trust the media to give you sound advice on how to lead a healthy, happy life? Consider the risks of blindly doing as you're told. Are more drugs, injections, and flu shots always the answer? On a scale of 1 to 10, how would you rate your level of Life Force Energy today?

NOTES:

DAY 11

UPON RISING: Dry brush thoroughly using your natural-bristle body brush, then devote some time to a body-enlivening activity of your choice.

PRE-BREAKFAST: Enjoy a minimum of eight to sixteen ounces of Life Force Power-ade or The Great Eliminator on an empty stomach.

BEFORE LEAVING HOME: Use the Life Force Power Breath for at least two full minutes (try it while tidying up your house—ah, the Zen of housekeeping!).

BREAKFAST: Enjoy any of the elixirs in the recipe section and/or fresh fruit as desired, stopping thirty minutes before your lunchtime meal.

LUNCH: Choose the most desirable option from pages 100–102 or a well-combined meal of your own. Have as much or as little as you need. While you're eating lunch, consider what you were taught about food as a child and how differently you understand nutrition now. You might try the Suddenly St. Tropez Salad (page 179) with some steamed vegetables and have any of the remaining raw goat cheese and veggies as a snack. Marinara sauce and Dijon mustard also make great nondense dips.

DINNER: Choose the most desirable dinner/dessert combination from pages 102–4 or a well-combined meal of your own. You might try the Don't Lose Your Cheesy Tacos (page 190) and the Raw Tomato Herb Potage with Shredded Raw Goat Cheese (page 169) and enjoy some dark chocolate for a dessert.

BEFORE RETIRING: Enjoy any evening activity of your choice—a massage, a hot bath, a walk, or meditation—that appeals to you. Be sure to make time to practice the Life Force Power Breath for five full, conscious minutes.

HOMEWORK: Meditate on these important elements in your life: Love, Praise, and Gratitude. As you do this, feel the vibrations in your body awakening and note how it feels. On a scale of 1 to 10, how would you rate your level of Life Force Energy today?

NOTES:

DAY 12

BEFORE RISING: Use the Life Force Power Breath for at least two full minutes—just lie there and breathe deeply as you anticipate the vibrant day ahead!

UPON RISING: Dry brush thoroughly with your natural-bristle body brush, then devote some time to a body-enlivening activity of your choice. Employ a gravity-method enema (or colonic) now or at some convenient time during the day when your stomach is empty.

PRE-BREAKFAST: Enjoy a minimum of eight to sixteen ounces of Life Force Power-ade or The Great Eliminator on an empty stomach.

BREAKFAST: Enjoy any of the elixirs in the recipe section and/or fresh fruit as desired, stopping thirty minutes before your lunchtime meal.

LUNCH: Choose the most desirable option from pages 100–102 or a well-combined meal of your own. Have as much or as little as you need. While you're eating lunch, think about how delicious natural foods are and how easy this program has become with practice!

You might try the Turkish Three-Pepper Tomato Salad (page 185) and the Raw Cream of Tomato Soup (page 167) and enjoy a couple of bananas or the Milk That Shakes & Shapes (page 223) for a snack at any time.

DINNER: Choose the most desirable dinner/dessert combination from pages 102–4 or a well-combined meal of your own. You might try the Parsnip-Carrot-Beet Bake (page 202), a sweet potato with greens, and sliced avocado topped with Quick

Balsamic Dressing (page 174), then enjoy an Organic Gourmet cookie or the Kollar cookies for a dessert.

BEFORE RETIRING: Enjoy any evening activity of your choice—a massage, a hot bath, a walk, or meditation—that appeals to you. Be sure to make time to practice the Life Force Power Breath for five full, conscious minutes.

HOMEWORK: Consider which body-opening activities you most enjoy. How can you make them even more fun?

On a scale of 1 to 10, how would you rate your level of Life Force Energy today?

NOTES:

DAY 13

UPON RISING: Dry brush thoroughly with your natural-bristle body brush, then devote some time to a body-enlivening activity of your choice.

PRE-BREAKFAST: Enjoy a minimum of twelve to twenty ounces of Life Force Power-ade or The Great Eliminator on an empty stomach.

BEFORE LEAVING HOME: Use the Life Force Power Breath for at least two full minutes (try it while reading your e-mails).

BREAKFAST: Enjoy any of the elixirs in the recipe section and/or fresh fruit as desired, stopping thirty minutes before your lunchtime meal.

LUNCH: Choose the most desirable option from pages 100–102 or a well-combined meal of your own. Have as much or as little as you need. While you're eating lunch, envision yourself a year from now continuing to live and eat this way. Imagine the strides you will have made in your health and appearance. You might try the Nut-Butter and Jelly Sandwiches (page 197) and your favorite raw vegetables or a simple salad, then have the Chocolate Mousse (page 223) or a Raw Bakery brownie for a snack anytime.

DINNER: Choose the most desirable dinner/dessert combination from pages 102–4 or a well-combined meal of your own. You might try the Powerful Beet-Parsley Cleansing Salad (page 184) and Pumpkin Pie in a Bowl (page 166), then enjoy some young coconut flesh and/or a few dates for dessert.

BEFORE RETIRING: Enjoy any evening activity of your choice—a massage, a hot bath, a walk, or meditation—that appeals to you. Be sure to make time to practice the Life Force Power Breath for five full, conscious minutes.

HOMEWORK: Treat yourself to a professional massage—preferably one that integrates acupressure points and/or chakra balancing, if you can find it.

On a scale of 1 to 10, how would you rate your level of Life Force Energy today?

NOTES:

DAY 14

UPON RISING: Dry brush thoroughly with your natural-bristle body brush, then devote some time to a body-enlivening activity of your choice.

PRE-BREAKFAST: Enjoy a minimum of twelve to twenty ounces of Life Force Power-ade or The Great Eliminator on an empty stomach.

BEFORE LEAVING HOME: Use the Life Force Power Breath for at least three full minutes (try it cross-legged like a yogi).

BREAKFAST: Enjoy any of the elixirs in the recipe section and/or fresh fruit as desired, stopping thirty minutes before your lunchtime meal.

LUNCH: Choose the most desirable option from pages 100–102 or a well-combined meal of your own. Have as much or as little as you need. While you're eating lunch, consider how much more oxygenated your cells are now that you're putting all of the Raw Food Life Force Energy principles into action. You might try the Sun-Dried Summer Slimmer (page 182) and the Raw Tomato Herb Potage with Shredded Raw Goat Cheese (page 169), then have some of the raw goat cheese anytime later for a snack—I love it sliced thinly and rolled up in cabbage leaves with Dijon mustard! Or if you prefer, you can have some fresh fruit three hours later.

DINNER: Choose the most desirable dinner/dessert combination from pages 102–4 or a well-combined meal of your own. You might try the Daily Avocado Classic (page 180) with Parsnip-Carrot-Beet Bake (page 202) and enjoy a high-quality whole-grain cookie or a couple of slices of sprouted-grain toast with raw honey for a dessert.

BEFORE RETIRING: Enjoy any evening activity of your choice—a massage, a hot bath, a walk, or meditation—that appeals to you. Be sure to make time to practice the Life Force Power Breath for five full, conscious minutes.

HOMEWORK: Go on an imaginary binge. Feel your stomach expanding, your consciousness diminishing, and your energy stagnating. Now reflect on your diet over the past two weeks—and the consequent feelings of lightness and vitality.

Take the Life Force Energy Body Test on page 109 again and see how you score has changed. Write your score here:_____

NOTES:

DAY 15

BEFORE RISING: Use the Life Force Power Breath for at least three full minutes. As you drink in the elixir of oxygen, set the intentions for your day and see them playing out as you would like.

PRE-BREAKFAST: Enjoy a minimum of twelve to twenty ounces of Life Force Power-ade or The Great Eliminator on an empty stomach.

BREAKFAST: Enjoy any of the elixirs in the recipe section and/or fresh fruit as desired, stopping thirty minutes before your lunchtime meal.

LUNCH: Choose the most desirable option from pages 100–102 or a well-combined meal of your own. Have as much or as little as you need. While you're eating lunch, consider how much more alive you feel throughout your whole body—as if you're on a natural high. You might try the Powerful Beet-Parsley Cleansing Salad (page 184) with The Best Thing Since Sliced Bread (page 218) and have some Ak-Mak crackers and your favorite raw vegetables anytime later as a snack.

DINNER: Choose the most desirable dinner/dessert combination from pages 102–4 or a well-combined meal of your own. You might try the Portobello-Marinara Grandwich (page 198) and the Sandwich Salad (page 186) and have some young coconut flesh or some dark chocolate for dessert.

BEFORE RETIRING: Enjoy one or more evening activity of your choice—a massage, a hot bath, a walk, or meditation—that appeals to you. Be sure to make time to practice the Life Force Power Breath for five full, conscious minutes.

HOMEWORK: Describe in as much detail as possible what it feels like physically and mentally when you tune into your energy field. On a scale of 1 to 10, how would you rate your level of Life Force Energy today?

NOTES:

DAY 16

UPON RISING: Dry brush thoroughly using your natural-bristle body brush, then devote some time to a body-enlivening activity of your choice.

PRE-BREAKFAST: Enjoy a minimum of twelve to twenty ounces of Life Force Power-ade or The Great Eliminator on an empty stomach.

BEFORE LEAVING HOME: Use the Life Force Power Breath for at least three full minutes (try it while in deep stretch positions or during a brief cycle of yogic postures).

BREAKFAST: Enjoy any of the elixirs and/or fresh fruit as desired, stopping thirty minutes before your lunchtime meal.

LUNCH: Choose the most desirable option from pages 100–102 or a well-combined meal of your own. Have as much or as little as you need. While you're eating lunch, take a moment to be truly appreciative of the good things in your life. Note how good it feels to give thanks and invite more of that good energy into your life. Imagine sending waves of gratitude out into the universe, to your family, your friends, and your acquaintances. You might try the Mega-Veggie Platter (page 206), a baked sweet potato, and simple greens with Quick Balsamic Dressing (page 174)—then enjoy your favorite whole-grain cookie or a young coconut as a snack or dessert. (The young coconut would be the more cleansing choice, of course. As a reminder, young coconuts combine well with everything except cheese and flesh, so there is no waiting time needed to enjoy the coconut following a starch meal such as this one.)

DINNER: Choose the most desirable dinner/dessert combination from pages 102–4 or a well-combined meal of your own. You might try the Raw Open-Faced

Sandwiches (page 197) and the Turkish Three-Pepper Tomato Salad (page 185), then have some dates or the Banana Cream Supreme Ice Cream (page 227) or the Milk That Shakes & Shapes (page 223) for dessert.

BEFORE RETIRING: Enjoy one or more evening activity of your choice—a massage, a hot bath, a walk, or meditation—that appeals to you. Be sure to make time to practice the Life Force Power Breath for five full, conscious minutes.

HOMEWORK: Describe in as much detail as possible how your body and mental state respond to Life Force Power Breath. On a scale of 1 to 10, how would you rate your level of Life Force Energy today?

NOTES:

DAY 17

UPON RISING: Dry brush thoroughly using your natural-bristle body brush, then devote some time to a body-enlivening exercise of your choice.

PRE-BREAKFAST: Enjoy a minimum of twelve to twenty ounces of Life Force Power-ade or The Great Eliminator on an empty stomach.

BEFORE LEAVING HOME: Use the Life Force Power Breath for at least three full minutes (try it while you're body brushing).

BREAKFAST: Enjoy any of the elixirs in the recipe section and/or fresh fruit as desired, stopping thirty minutes before your lunchtime meal.

LUNCH: Choose the most desirable option from pages 100–102 or a well-combined meal of your own. Have as much or as little as you need. While you're eating lunch, consider how your mood has changed over the past couple of weeks. You might try the Kombu Melt (page 208) and Sweet Basil Tomato Towers (page 207), and have some of the goat cheese left over from the Kombu Melt and/or some dark chocolate as a dessert or snack.

DINNER: Choose the most desirable dinner/dessert combination from pages 102–4 or a well-combined meal of your own. You might try the Salad Sandwich (page 200) and the Cleansing Corn Chowder (page 168) and have a few ears of corn and your favorite raw vegetables with some homemade guacamole anytime for a snack.

BEFORE RETIRING: Enjoy one or more evening activity of your choice—a massage, a hot bath, a walk, or meditation—that appeals to you. Be sure to make time to practice the Life Force Power Breath for five full, conscious minutes.

HOMEWORK: Write down what it feels like to have Life Force Energy flowing through your body. How would you describe it? On a scale of 1 to 10, how would you rate your level of Life Force Energy today?

NOTES:

DAY 18

UPON RISING: Dry brush thoroughly using your natural-bristle body brush, then devote some time to a body-enlivening activity of your choice.

PRE-BREAKFAST: Enjoy a minimum of twelve to twenty ounces of Life Force Power-ade or The Great Eliminator on an empty stomach.

BEFORE LEAVING HOME: Use the Life Force Power Breath for at least three full minutes.

BREAKFAST: Enjoy any of the elixirs in the recipe section and/or fresh fruit as desired, stopping thirty minutes before your lunchtime meal.

LUNCH: Choose the most desirable option from pages 100–102 or a well-combined meal of your own. Have as much or as little as you need. While you're eating lunch, imagine every cell in your body dancing with vitality. You might try the Pineapple's Just Peachy Summer Soup (page 171) with the Raw Open-Faced Sandwiches (page 197) and have the Chocolate Mousse (page 223) or a couple of bananas anytime as a snack.

DINNER: Choose the most desirable dinner/dessert combination from pages 102–4 or a well-combined meal of your own. You might try the Age of Aquarius Mac 'n' Cheese (page 205) and the Summer Salad, Poolside (page 183) with some dark chocolate for dessert.

BEFORE RETIRING: Enjoy one or more evening activity of your choice—a massage, a hot bath, a walk, or meditation—that appeals to you. Be sure to make time to practice the Life Force Power Breath for five full, conscious minutes.

HOMEWORK: Write down your deepest regrets, disappointments, and resentments. Can you explain to yourself how keeping these in your heart and mind will improve your life? If you cannot find a good reason to hold onto them, imagine letting them go one by one. Now write down your greatest joys and how keeping them in your heart and mind will improve your life. On a scale of 1 to 10, how would you rate your level of Life Force Energy today?

NOTES:

DAY 19

UPON RISING: Dry brush thoroughly using your natural-bristle body brush, then devote some time to a body-enlivening activity of your choice.

PRE-BREAKFAST: Enjoy a minimum of twelve to twenty ounces of Life Force Power-ade or The Great Eliminator on an empty stomach.

BEFORE LEAVING HOME: Use the Life Force Power Breath for at least three full minutes (try it while you're preparing fresh fruits for breakfast at home or to take to the office).

BREAKFAST: Enjoy any of the elixirs in the recipe section and/or fresh fruit as desired, stopping thirty minutes before your lunchtime meal.

LUNCH: Choose the most desirable option from pages 100–102 or a well-combined meal of your own. Have as much or as little as you need. While you're eating lunch, consider what an important role the Life Force Power-ade has played in this program and remind yourself to do it long after you've completed these 21 days. You might try a basic tossed salad (any mix of raw vegetables with balsamic- or lemon juice–based dressing), a baked sweet potato, and several Ak-Mak crackers, then enjoy some raw sliced vegetables and guacamole dip anytime thereafter as a snack. Or wait three hours and enjoy some fresh fruit or your favorite freshly extracted vegetable juice.

DINNER: Choose the most desirable dinner/dessert combination from pages 102–4 or a well-combined meal of your own. You might try your favorite fish dish along with your favorite raw vegetable salad and dark chocolate for dessert.

BEFORE RETIRING: Enjoy one or more evening activity of your choice—a massage, a hot bath, a walk, or meditation—that appeals to you. Be sure to make time to practice the Life Force Power Breath for five full, conscious minutes.

HOMEWORK: Write down your experience with colon cleansing. How did it make you feel afterward? Will you continue to have colon cleansings after this 21-day program? Write down whether you felt safe and whether the experience made sense to you and harmonized with your body. On a scale of 1 to 10, how would you rate your level of Life Force Energy today?

NOTES:

DAY 20

UPON RISING: Dry brush thoroughly using your natural-bristle body brush, then devote some time to a body-enlivening activity of your choice.

PRE-BREAKFAST: Enjoy a minimum of twelve to twenty ounces of Life Force Power-ade or The Great Eliminator on an empty stomach.

BEFORE LEAVING HOME: Use the Life Force Power Breath for at least three full minutes (try it while you're paying your bills or sorting through your mail).

BREAKFAST: Enjoy any of the elixirs in the recipe section and/or fresh fruit as desired, stopping thirty minutes before your lunchtime meal.

LUNCH: Choose the most desirable option from pages 100–102 or a well-combined meal of your own. Have as much or as little as you need. While you're eating lunch, think about how you will continue using the practical applications in this book; getting your groceries; making your juice; making high-vibration, high–Life Force Energy recipes; and staying motivated after tomorrow. You might try the Nut-Butter and Jelly Sandwiches (page 197) with some fresh raw greens (dressed simply with fresh lemon juice and stevia or agave nectar) followed up anytime with a scoop of Banana Cream Supreme Ice Cream (page 227).

DINNER: Choose the most desirable dinner/dessert combination from pages 102–4 or a well-combined meal of your own. You might try the Herb-Encrusted Swordfish (page 213) and Turkish Three-Pepper Tomato Salad (page 185) and enjoy some of the dark chocolate for dessert.

BEFORE RETIRING: Enjoy one or more evening activity of your choice—a massage, a hot bath, a walk, or meditation—that appeals to you. Be sure to make time to practice the Life Force Power Breath for five full, conscious minutes.

HOMEWORK: Do you hold a particular grudge against someone in your life? Do you wish to be connected to that person in this way? Now imagine that positive energy is trying to reach you, but it cannot because all of this negative energy is in its way. Visualize cutting this negative cord and setting yourself free from it. Summon full forgiveness so that good feelings can flow into your energy field without impediment. Visualize abundance for yourself and that person you set free. Do this exercise again and again for every person you need to forgive—including yourself. On a scale of 1 to 10, how would you rate your level of Life Force Energy today?

NOTES:

DAY 21

BEFORE RISING: Use the Life Force Power Breath for at least three full minutes (try it while thinking only of each inhalation and exhalation).

UPON RISING: Dry brush thoroughly using your natural-bristle body brush, then devote some time to a body-enlivening activity of your choice. Employ a gravity-method enema (or colonic) now or at some convenient time during the day when your stomach is empty.

PRE-BREAKFAST: Enjoy a minimum of twelve to twenty ounces of Life Force Power-ade or The Great Eliminator on an empty stomach.

BREAKFAST: Fresh fruit as desired, stopping thirty minutes before your lunchtime meal.

LUNCH: Choose the most desirable option from pages 100–102 or a well-combined meal of your own. Have as much or as little as you need. While you're eating lunch, consider the difference between the "old you" who started this program 21 days ago and the "new you" today. You might try the Sweet Potato Beet Pasta with Pesto and Diced Tomatoes (page 191) and have several slices of The Best Thing Since Sliced Bread (page 218) as a snack.

DINNER: Choose the most desirable dinner/dessert combination from pages 102–4 or a well-combined meal of your own. You might try the Daily Avocado Classic (page 180) with the Parsnip-Carrot-Beet Bake (page 202) and enjoy your favorite whole-grain cookie(s) for dessert.

BEFORE RETIRING: Enjoy one or more evening activity of your choice—a massage, a hot bath, a walk, or meditation—that appeals to you. Be sure to make time to practice the Life Force Power Breath for five full, conscious minutes.

HOMEWORK: Write down your physical experience today and compare it to your physical experience on Day 1. Now write down what you plan to do with this new perspective. Visualize your body and your mental/spiritual state growing more beautiful and joyful for years to come. Picture yourself one year from now, ten years from now, thirty years from now . . . looking and feeling ever more connected, centered, and attractive! On a scale of 1 to 10, how would you rate your level of Life

Force Energy today? Take the Life Force Energy Body Test on page 109 again and see how your score has changed. Write your score here:

NOTES:

I recommend that you save all your notes and reflections from this 21-day program and let them serve as a reminder of the wonderful metamorphosis you've experienced over the last three weeks. They will come in handy in numerous ways: first, if you ever fall back into your old patterns, your notes will remind you how much the program did for your body and your headspace in a short period of time; second, seeing just how far you've come from your old habits will help keep you motivated to stay the course; and finally, one day you'll be able to appreciate the long-term cumulative effects of this program, which is where its true power really lies.

It's fun to look back on these logs. I recommend that you continue to keep some sort of journal to follow your progress beyond these initial 21 days, even if you log in only a couple times a week. Keep a section called "What I'm eating now" to record the foods and food combinations that you enjoy on a regular basis. They will likely change with each season, and as the years go by you can glance back to recall what you enjoyed during a previous season whenever you're feeling short on ideas. And if you follow the Raw Food Life Force Energy program with friends, you can share your logs and help inspire each other!

PART III

RAW FOOD LIFE FORCE ENERGY RECIPES

WELCOME TO THE WORLD OF RAW FOOD ENERGY CUISINE!

You are going to love the following recipes, which are overflowing with flavor and vitality. Sharpen your knives and whet your appetite with a great big Life Force Energy Power Breath and let's get started!

To help you create quick-exit meal combinations, the food category each recipe falls under is written below the recipe name. Keep in mind the simple rule of quick-exit food combining: *Like categories mix with like categories and all neutral items.* I cannot stress enough how this single rule can radically improve your shape and energy level! At the same time, for those of you who are just beginning to transition into this diet lifestyle and simply want to feel better eating natural foods, these recipes will benefit you tremendously even if you don't pay a lot of attention to food combining. In other words, the more you adhere to proper food combining, the more effective the program will be, but these foods are so clean and life generating that even without strict adherence to quick-exit combinations you should see great results!

RAW FOOD LIFE FORCE ENERGY RECIPE LIST

ELIXIRS

The elixirs are deeply hydrating, oxygen-rich liquids—the most perfect drinks for the Life Force Energy seeker. Enjoy them as often as you like, in larger or smaller quantities based on your needs. Feel free to play around with the ingredients as well, making the recipes your own.

Since the life force of freshly juiced produce peaks the moment it is made, try not to leave it too long before drinking. If you'd like it to keep, you may freeze it. I often freeze my juice in preparation for long trips so that the day I travel, the juice will be freshly defrosted several hours into my journey when I need it most but cannot prepare it.

When juicing, use organic fruits and vegetables whenever possible. It is more important to use organic vegetables for juicing than for other recipes, as juicing requires a much larger quantity of produce.

Depending on your juicer, you may need to cut your produce into pieces that will fit through the nozzle. Any juicer will do, but I recommend the juicers made by Breville (whichever model fits best into your budget—they are all good). They are surprisingly easy to use and clean, which is key to ensuring long-term use.

LIFE FORCE POWER-ADE

Enjoy only on an empty stomach.

MAKES 3 TO 4 CUPS

6 to 8 leaves fresh kale with stems

2 apples (use more or less as desired for taste)

1 whole lemon with peel

1 whole medium-sized beet

1 head celery or 2 cucumbers

1 to 2 tablespoons fresh ginger (optional)

Put each ingredient one at a time through the mouth of a high-powered juicer. Pour the juice into a large glass and enjoy!

Note: Stevia may be substituted in place of the apple to sweeten if you are avoiding fruit for any reason.

THE GREAT ELIMINATOR

Enjoy only on an empty stomach.

MAKES 2 TO 3 CUPS

1 medium or large beet

1 cucumber

10 medium-sized carrots

1 inch fresh ginger (optional)

Put each ingredient one at a time through the mouth of a high-powered juicer. Pour the juice into a large glass and enjoy!

CLEANSING WATERMELON COCKTAIL

Best on an empty stomach or with fresh fruit.

MAKES 5 TO 6 CUPS

¼ **whole watermelon**

1 **lime with peel**

1 **inch fresh ginger**

Wash the watermelon rind well, then slice the watermelon into pieces suitable for your high-powered juicer. Put each ingredient one at a time through the mouth of the juicer. Serve in martini glasses as a cocktail anytime. Sure beats a Bloody Mary for Sunday brunch!

CHIA-A WAWA

Neutral. This simple drink is incredibly complex in flavor. It will revive and hydrate you more than any caffeinated beverage. Try it in the morning before work, after a long day, or on a hot summer afternoon and see for yourself how it revives and delights!

MAKES 2 CUPS

2 **cups fresh, young coconut water (see note below)**

¼ **teaspoon Indian chai spice blend (can be found at any health food or Indian store)**

Pour coconut water into a glass or a blender, add the chai spice, and either blend or shake for several seconds.

Note: Use water from 1 to 2 fresh young coconuts, not from canned coconut cream or packaged coconut water of any kind. If you don't want to open them yourself with a cleaver, ask the market to open them for you and place the "water" in a travel-friendly container.

FRESH MINT ELIXIR

Neutral

This is a great drink to keep in the fridge for guests. It becomes more flavorful over the course of a day. It's refreshing and leaves everyone feeling clean and high-vibing!

MAKES ABOUT 9 CUPS

64 ounces fresh water

½ medium cucumber, sliced into thin disks

1 to 3 sprigs fresh mint

1 medium carrot, sliced into thin disks

1 lemon, sliced into thin disks

Mix all ingredients in a large jug or pitcher. Stir and enjoy throughout the day.

ORANGE ZEST

Neutral

This is the drink I recommend most to people who are trying to stop drinking sodas and feel the need for something other than water. It's charged with electrolytes from the citrus, deeply hydrating, and also sweet—essentially a fresh fruit juice–infused water.

MAKES ABOUT 8 CUPS

> **64 ounces purified water**
>
> **1 whole lemon, sliced**
>
> **1 whole orange, sliced**
>
> **1 to 3 sprigs fresh mint**
>
> **1 lime, sliced**
>
> **3 packets Stevia**

Mix all ingredients into a large jug or pitcher. Stir and enjoy throughout the day.

THE OXYGENATOR

Neutral, but best on an empty stomach

This elixir is great for increasing circulation. Enjoy the feeling of warmth as the ginger and chilies work to remove the blockages to your Life Force Energy. The beet will encourage bowel elimination and the sweetness of the carrots will soften the taste of the ginger and cayenne pepper, making for a smooth, pleasurable beverage.

MAKES ABOUT 2½ CUPS

> **1 pound carrots**
>
> **1 medium-sized beet**
>
> **1 tablespoon fresh ginger**
>
> **¼ teaspoon ground cayenne pepper or fresh Serrano chili**

Put each ingredient one at a time through the mouth of a high-powered juicer. Pour the juice into a large glass and enjoy!

HOLIDAY ANYTIME

Neutral, but like all vegetable juices, best on an empty stomach

The rich combination of pumpkin pie spice and milky carrot juice is a taste that anyone will love—kids included! Yet it's as pure as simple, fresh carrot juice. The nutmeg, clove, and cinnamon in the pumpkin pie spice blend has a warming effect and, I find, is most delightful when served in a mug!

MAKES 2 CUPS

> **16 ounces fresh carrot juice**
>
> **¼ tablespoon pumpkin pie spice**

Place both ingredients in a blender or a large mug and mix for just a few seconds.

GREEN JUICE IN A PINCH

Enjoy only on an empty stomach

I created this juice one day when I came home after a long day of work, feeling too exhausted even to wait for a delivery of fresh green vegetable juice from my local health food store. I remembered that I had some frozen wheatgrass cubes and whipped this number up. To my delight, it gave me the lift I needed and tasted great, too!

MAKES ABOUT 2 CUPS

> **4 cubes frozen organic wheatgrass (I use the Evergreen brand, which is available in the freezer at most health food stores)**
>
> **1 to 2 bags of your favorite herbal tea (I recommend mint or orange)**
>
> **3 packets Stevia**
>
> **Juice of half a lemon**

Place all of the ingredients in a large mug or glass. Pour 1½ cups of warm water (not hot) over the mixture. Let the frozen wheatgrass cubes melt, and then stir the mixture.

KOMBUCHA DIGESTIF

Neutral, but best on an empty stomach*

Kombucha is a Chinese tea that is cultured to form probiotics, which support the regeneration of good bacteria in the intestines.

MAKES 1 CUP

> **1 cup of Synergy grape-flavored kombucha (available in the refrigerator at most health food stores)**
>
> **Juice of half a lemon**
>
> **2 packets Stevia**

Mix all of the ingredients in a glass and enjoy.

> *You can combine this drink with all other foods if you like, but to benefit from the natural bacteria you must consume it on an empty stomach.*

SOUPS

Some of these soups are 100 percent *live* and uncooked, and others are heated. The raw soups are great for lunch or as a part of an all-raw dinner. The cooked soups make a great, hot meal by themselves or as part of a raw and/or cooked dinner. All of the soups are very easy to digest and therefore help to increase the flow of Life Force Energy!

PUMPKIN PIE IN A BOWL

Raw, avocado-based

This is among the recipes that I'm most excited to share with you. Why? Because this utterly delicious soup provides tons of live enzymes in an incredibly digestible form. Neither my clients nor I can get enough of it. It's all raw, and it supports weight loss and vitality, so enjoy *as much of it as you like* as part of a meal or as a snack.

I found that it's best to double the recipe when I plan on having more than one or two guests. It may look like a lot, but this soup is so good that you might eat most of it before your guests even arrive!

MAKES 5½ CUPS

4 cups fresh carrot juice

1 cup raw sweet potato, peeled and cubed

4 dates, pitted

½ avocado, pitted

½ teaspoon pumpkin pie spice

Place all of the ingredients in a high-speed blender and blend until smooth. Enjoy right away or store in an air-tight container and enjoy within 36 hours.

RAW CREAM OF TOMATO SOUP

Raw, avocado-based

This soup is so light and fresh that you may enjoy as much as you like.

MAKES ABOUT 3 CUPS

> **4 to 5 fresh, fragrant tomatoes (I recommend Holland or Roma), quartered**
>
> **¼ cup cilantro**
>
> **1 avocado, pitted and scooped out**
>
> **1 packet Stevia**
>
> **1 teaspoon agave nectar (the sweet substance derived from the cactus plant)**
>
> **Sea salt and fresh pepper to taste**
>
> **½ cup apple, chopped (see note)**
>
> **½ cup fresh corn off the cob (see note)**

In a mixing bowl, blend all of the ingredients, except the apple and the corn, until creamy. In a separate bowl, mix the chopped apple and corn kernels together, then divide the corn-apple mixture between two serving bowls. Ladle the soup over the mixture in each bowl and serve.

Note: You may enjoy this soup with or without the corn-apple mixture.

CLEANSING CORN CHOWDER

Raw, avocado-based

"Cleansing Corn Chowder" may sound like an oxymoron, but this raw version is both hearty and light!

MAKES 6 TO 7 CUPS

> **4 cups corn off the cob (about 4 to 5 large ears)**
>
> **2 cups Pacific brand almond milk (see note)**
>
> **1 avocado**
>
> **1 teaspoon cumin**
>
> **2 teaspoons finely minced onion**
>
> **Celtic sea salt and fresh ground black pepper to taste**
>
> **¼ cup alfalfa sprouts (optional)**
>
> **¼ cup diced red bell pepper (optional)**

Setting aside about ¼ cup of the corn, the sprouts, and the bell pepper, blend the rest of the ingredients together well in a mixing bowl. Plate the mixture and top with a sprinkling of reserved corn kernels, the sprouts, and/or the diced red pepper bits as desired.

> *Note: If you prefer, you can make your own almond milk by blending 1 cup of almonds with 3 cups of water in a blender and straining the mixture through a cheese cloth or a very fine sieve to separate the liquid from the pulp, which gets discarded.*

RAW TOMATO HERB POTAGE WITH SHREDDED RAW GOAT CHEESE

Flesh category*

MAKES 2 SERVINGS

5 Roma or Holland tomatoes, diced

4 sun-dried tomatoes, soaked in warm water until soft and diced

¼ cup chopped fresh basil leaves

Sea salt and fresh pepper to taste

1 clove garlic, diced

2 tablespoons finely chopped fresh oregano

½ cup shredded raw cheddar-style goat cheese (I recommend Alta Dena, but Shiloh Farms or any other brand will do)

In a large bowl, mix together all of the ingredients except the shredded cheese. Distribute evenly into two soup bowls and top with the shredded cheese. Serve at room temperature or slightly warmed.

Remember, cheese falls under the "flesh" category. While it is not literally a flesh food, it mixes best as such, going perfectly with vegetables and other flesh category items.

GRAIN-FREE ASIAN KOMBU NOODLE SOUP

Neutral

This is a great cold weather soup. It really heats you up inside.

MAKES ABOUT 5 CUPS OR 4 SERVINGS

> 3 cups organic vegetable broth
>
> 1 cup julienned carrots
>
> 1 cup thinly sliced Lotus root
>
> 1 cup sliced shiitake mushrooms
>
> 1 tablespoon minced fresh ginger
>
> 1 tablespoon minced fresh garlic
>
> 1 tablespoon soy sauce (the Nama Shoyu brand, if possible)
>
> 1 tablespoon red miso paste
>
> 1 teaspoon sesame oil (toasted, if desired)
>
> 2 packets soft Kombu seaweed noodles, rinsed (see note)
>
> ½ cup snow pea shoots (available in most gourmet stores and farmers markets, but if you cannot find them, they may be omitted)

In a large soup pot, combine all of the ingredients except the the Kombu noodles and the snow pea shoots. Bring ingredients to a boil and let simmer for about 10 minutes. Ladle the soup mixture evenly on top of the Kombu noodles in a large serving bowl. Dress with the snow pea shoots.

Note: If you cannot find Kombu seaweed noodles easily at your health food or gourmet grocery, you may order them online at www.kombu-noodle.com. This particular brand is soft and pasta-like, packed in water and ready to use.

PINEAPPLE'S JUST PEACHY SUMMER SOUP

Fresh fruit category

MAKES ABOUT 2 SERVINGS

> **1 cup chopped pineapple**
>
> **2 peaches, sliced**
>
> **½ cup sliced strawberries**
>
> **½ cup fresh raspberries**
>
> **½ cup packed alfalfa sprouts**
>
> **2 tablespoons agave nectar**
>
> **1 teaspoon balsamic vinegar**
>
> **¼ teaspoon diced Serrano chili**
>
> **4 sprigs of mint**

In a blender, mix all of the ingredients, except the balsamic vinegar and the chili, and blend until smooth. In a small bowl, toss the balsamic vinegar with the chili and sprinkle on top of the soup. Dress with the sprigs of mint.

SENSEI SAID SOBA NOODLE SOUP

Starch

MAKES 4 TO 6 SERVINGS

- 1 package soba noodles, cooked in boiling water until soft (about 5 minutes)

- ½ cup shiitake mushrooms

- ½ cup snow pea shoots (available at most gourmet stores year round)

- ½ cup sugar snap peas

- 1 cup chopped carrots

- ¼ cup chopped fresh cilantro

- 1 tablespoon soy sauce or Nama Shoyu (raw soy sauce)

- ¼ cup reconstituted seaweed of choice (I'd recommend arame or nori strips)

- ½ cup mung bean sprouts

- 4 cups Pacific brand organic vegetable broth

- 1 tablespoon diced fresh ginger

- 1 clove garlic, diced

In a soup pot, mix all of the ingredients, except the noodles, and cook on medium heat for about 12 minutes or until the carrots are tender. Cook the noodles until soft (about 6 to 8 minutes in boiling water) and rinse them well. Place the noodles in a bowl and ladle the soup mixture on top. Serve with chopsticks.

DRESSINGS

When we start to build our diet around fresh produce, it's important to make the produce highly satisfying. A great dressing can transform an ordinary raw salad into a deeply satisfying meal. As you enjoy salads with these dressing, you will find that vegetables need not be boring or bland—quite the contrary! Dressings are the secret to making your vegetable salads something you can look forward to every day.

Each of the following dressings is light and delicious and requires very little effort to prepare. I recommend keeping a container of dressing wherever you eat—perhaps one at home and another one at your place of work so that you can always dress some raw vegetables or greens for a delicious, satisfying snack or meal.

SWEET CHILI-LIME DRESSING

Neutral

MAKES 1½ TO 2 CUPS

> 1 cup fresh-squeezed lime juice
>
> 4 packets Stevia
>
> ¼ cup agave nectar
>
> 1 teaspoon minced Serrano chili
>
> 1 tablespoon chopped garlic
>
> Salt and pepper to taste
>
> ¼ cup cold-pressed olive oil

Blend all of the ingredients, except the oil, until smooth. Then blend in the oil a little at a time to emulsify it and keep it from separating. Keeps in the refrigerator for up to 2 weeks.

QUICK BALSAMIC DRESSING

Neutral

MAKES 1½ CUPS

> 1 cup balsamic vinegar
>
> 5 packets Stevia
>
> 1 tablespoon chopped garlic
>
> Celtic sea salt and fresh pepper to taste
>
> ¼ cup cold-pressed olive oil

Blend all of the ingredients, except the oil, until smooth. Then blend in the oil a little at a time to emulsify it and keep it from separating. Keeps in the refrigerator for up to 2 weeks.

SESAME GINGERSNAP DRESSING

Neutral

MAKES 1 TO 1½ CUPS

- 1 clove garlic
- 1 tablespoon minced fresh ginger
- 2 tablespoons agave nectar
- 2 tablespoons apple juice
- 2 packets Stevia
- ¼ cup cold-pressed olive oil
- ½ cup unpasteurized grapefruit juice
- Celtic sea salt and pepper to taste

Blend all of the ingredients, except the oil, until smooth. Then blend in the oil a little at a time to emulsify it and keep it from separating. Keeps in the refrigerator for 1 to 2 weeks.

RASPBERRY-LIME TART DRESSING

Neutral*

MAKES ABOUT 1½ CUPS

> ½ cup fresh raspberries
>
> ½ cup fresh squeezed lime juice
>
> 5 packets Stevia
>
> ¼ cup pure maple syrup or agave nectar
>
> Celtic sea salt and fresh pepper to taste

Blend all ingredients until smooth. Keeps in the refrigerator for about 3 days.

> *Because there is so little fruit in this recipe per serving, it may be treated as neutral.*

RASPBERRY-BALSAMIC DRESSING

Neutral*

MAKES ABOUT 1½ CUPS

> ½ cup fresh raspberries
>
> ¼ cup balsamic vinegar
>
> 5 packets Stevia
>
> ¼ cup pure maple syrup or agave nectar
>
> Salt and pepper to taste

Blend all ingredients until smooth. Keeps in the refrigerator for about 3 days.

> *Because there is so little fruit in this recipe per serving, it may be treated as neutral.*

CREAMY HERB LIVE YOGURT DRESSING

Flesh category

MAKES ABOUT 1½ CUPS

> 1 cup raw goat milk yogurt
>
> 3 tablespoons raw honey or agave nectar (or 2 packets NuNaturals brand Stevia)
>
> 1 teaspoon chopped rosemary
>
> 1 teaspoon chopped chives
>
> ¼ cup fresh lemon juice

Blend all ingredients until smooth. Keeps in the refrigerator for 3 to 5 days.

SALADS

Salads take on a whole new meaning in this diet-lifestyle. They are neither a small appetizer nor a mixed meal of everything in sight tossed together. For this diet-lifestyle, salads are carefully combined centerpieces that are so succulent and flavorful that they usually become our favorite meals. You may enjoy every one of these salads as a completely satisfying entrée (simply double the portion) or as a delicious appetizer. Each recipe is an ideal choice for a lunch meal.

As you develop your salad-making skills, you will gain a whole new appreciation for salads. These recipes will allow you to please your palate, nourish and heal your body, and increase your flow of Life Force Energy every day.

SUDDENLY ST. TROPEZ

Flesh category

This is the salad I eat more often than any other. I love the way the balsamic vinegar, Stevia, and grated goat cheese come together so decadently while the greens and tomatoes keep the whole dish tasting fresh from the garden. The beets offer a colorful twist, reminiscent of the great beet and goat cheese salads at the best French bistros. For a simpler dish, try this recipe without the optional herbs and onion. For a showpiece, add everything. There is no oil in this salad because it's best to avoid doubling up on fats for easy digestion. Cheese is the fat ingredient in this recipe, so we can omit the oil and still balance out the acidity from the balsamic vinegar.

MAKES 2 TO 4 SERVINGS

¼ to ½ pounds mesclun or baby romaine lettuce

1 cup grape tomatoes, halved

1 medium beet, peeled and finely julienned into spaghetti-like strips

3 ounces Alta Dena raw cheddar-style goat cheese, grated

2 to 3 tablespoons balsamic vinegar

3 to 4 packets Stevia

1 tablespoon diced fresh garlic

Sea salt and fresh pepper to taste

2 tablespoons diced sweet onion (optional)

¼ cup chopped fresh basil (optional)

2 tablespoons chopped fresh oregano or chives (optional)

Toss all of the ingredients together in a large salad bowl and serve.

DAILY AVOCADO CLASSIC

Raw, avocado-based

The simple, savory sweetness of a creamy avocado mixed with Stevia and balsamic vinegar is the ultimate, easy gourmet concoction. Add more avocado to this salad if you'd like it heartier. The more you mix it up, the creamier it gets. In this salad, the avocado is the fat ingredient, so no oil is required.

MAKES 2 TO 4 SERVINGS

> ¼ to ½ pound mesclun or baby romaine lettuce
>
> 1 ripe avocado, chopped
>
> 1 cup grape tomatoes, halved
>
> 2 to 3 tablespoons balsamic vinegar
>
> 3 to 4 packets Stevia
>
> 1 tablespoon diced fresh garlic
>
> Sea salt and fresh pepper to taste
>
> 2 tablespoons diced sweet onion (optional)

Toss all of the ingredients together in a large salad bowl and serve.

SALAD GONE NUTS

Raw, nut based

The candied almonds in this recipe are dehydrated at low temperatures to preserve their live enzymes. Their flavor is out of this world! The Almond Brothers brand offers many different nuts and flavors to choose from. I also highly recommend the chili-pistachios. You can order them online at www.therawfooddetoxdiet.com. Almond Brothers produces the most delicious, high-quality candied, curried, and spiced varieties of your favorite nuts—all protected from heating over 118 degrees to offer a true delicacy with no loss of Life Force Energy!

MAKES 2 SERVINGS

¼ to ½ **pound mesclun or baby romaine lettuce**

1 cup grape tomatoes, halved

¼ **cup grated or julienned carrots**

¼ **cup candied almonds or other dehydrated nuts by Almond Brothers**

3 tablespoons raisins

2 to 3 tablespoons balsamic vinegar

3 to 4 packets Stevia

1 tablespoon diced fresh garlic

Sea salt and fresh pepper to taste

2 tablespoons diced sweet onion (optional)

Mix all of the ingredients together in a big salad bowl and serve.

SUN-DRIED SUMMER SLIMMER

Flesh category

This recipe is the closest I have come to mimicking the flavor of pizza in a salad.

MAKES 2 SERVINGS

> 6 to 8 unsulfured sun-dried tomatoes, soaked in lukewarm water until soft, chopped
>
> ¼ to ½ pound fresh baby greens
>
> 3 ounces Alta Dena or Shiloh Farms raw cheddar-style goat cheese, shredded
>
> ¼ cup chopped fresh basil
>
> 1 tablespoon chopped oregano
>
> 1 tablespoon balsamic vinegar
>
> 2 packets Stevia
>
> 1 clove garlic, chopped (optional)
>
> Sea salt and pepper to taste

Mix all of the ingredients together and devour!

SUMMER SALAD, POOLSIDE

Raw, avocado based

MAKES 1 TO 2 SERVINGS

- **2 ounces fresh arugula or spinach**
- **1 avocado, sliced**
- **1 bulb fennel, julienned**
- **½ cup sweet cherry tomatoes, halved**
- **1 orange bell pepper, julienned**
- **¼ cup sliced scallions**
- **2 to 3 tablespoons of Quick Balsamic Dressing (page 174), or more as desired**
- **1 tablespoon fresh dill (optional)**
- **1 tablespoon finely chopped fresh rosemary (optional)**

Plate all of the vegetables artfully, mixing up the colors, and top with the dressing and the herbs.

POWERFUL BEET-PARSLEY CLEANSING SALAD BY IBRAHIM "IBO" GENCAY OF THE RAW BAKERY

Neutral

Ibo Gencay is the executive chef and CEO of The Raw Bakery, a leading raw food company that produces some of the best premade raw food items available. I highly recommend checking out The Raw Bakery goods, particularly their brownies and macaroons! You can order them from www.rawbakery.com or by calling 1-800-571-8369. The products are also sold at many health food stores.

In Ibo's own words, "Eat this when you feel like you want some nutrients from the earth. Beets and carrots grow below the ground and supply you with an abundance of minerals. Imagine the colorful red beet inside your body and what it will do for you."

MAKES 2 SERVINGS

2 medium-sized beets, peeled and grated

4 medium-sized carrots, grated

½ bunch curled or flat leaf parsley, minced

3 medium-sized tomatoes or 4 plum tomatoes, diced

2 to 3 tablespoons cold-pressed extra virgin olive oil

1½ tablespoons fresh-squeezed lemon juice

½ teaspoon sea salt

½ teaspoon ground black pepper

Mix all of the ingredients together in a large salad bowl. Let the salad sit and marinate in its juices for at least a few minutes before serving.

TURKISH THREE-PEPPER TOMATO SALAD BY IBRAHIM "IBO" GENCAY OF THE RAW BAKERY

Neutral

The master raw food chef tells me that this is the salad he makes most often. It is quick and easy to prepare, and tastes divine!

MAKES 2 SERVINGS

2 green peppers, diced

2 red peppers, diced

1 yellow or orange pepper

10 Roma tomatoes, diced

⅓ cup diced red or white onion

3 tablespoons cold-pressed, extra virgin olive oil

2 tablespoons fresh-squeezed lemon juice

1 teaspoon sea salt

½ to 1 teaspoon ground black pepper

Mix all ingredients in a large salad bowl.

SANDWICH SALAD

Raw, avocado-based

This salad has all the fixings of a vegetable sandwich in salad form. I came up with this recipe when I caught the fresh scent of the sprout and vegetable sandwich that my husband was eating one day. I realized the blissful fragrance had nothing to do with the bread and everything to do with the onions, parsley, and Dijon!

MAKES 2 SERVINGS

¼ cup alfalfa sprouts

1 red or orange bell pepper, julienned

¼ medium cucumber, thinly sliced

½ avocado, sliced

1 tablespoon finely chopped parsley

1 tablespoon finely chopped cilantro

1 tablespoon Dijon mustard

Spike seasoning to taste (a must-have, all-purpose herbal seasoning, which is available at any health food store)

Mix together all of the ingredients in a salad bowl and serve.

RAW ENTRÉES

The raw entrées are great for lunches and dinners—either alone or combined properly with other recipes. Their novelty, beautiful colors, tantalizing fragrances, and wonderful flavors make them great dishes for entertaining.

Some of the raw entrées, such as the taco and spaghetti dishes, are very easy to prepare but are just as delicious and filling as the more complex dishes. Such dishes as Sushi to Impress and the raviolis will naturally appeal to those who are inclined to invest more effort into creating innovative raw meals.

There have been times when I've wanted to try every raw food recipe, regardless of the amount of preparation, and other times when I've wanted all the flavor and fullness without investing in it more than five or ten minutes. These recipes are for chefs of all stages and skill levels.

SUSHI TO IMPRESS

Raw, avocado-based

MAKES 2 TO 4 SERVINGS

FOR THE CREAM FILLING:

1 medium avocado

¼ cup cubed carrots

1 clove fresh garlic, diced

1 teaspoon diced fresh ginger

1 tablespoon soy sauce (preferably Nama Shoyu)

1 tablespoon maple syrup

FOR THE VEGETABLE FILLING:

1 medium carrot, julienned

1 medium cucumber, julienned

1 red bell pepper, julienned

Snow pea shoots (if available at your local gourmet market or farm stand)

FOR THE "SUSHI RICE":

1 medium parsnip, chopped and pulsed in a food processor until it forms rice-like pieces

6 sheets nori (seaweed)

1. Blend the ingredients for the cream filling in a food processor until smooth.

2. Place a sheet of nori on a wooden cutting board so that the indented lines on the nori run horizontally. Place a thin layer of the cream filling on the lower third of the nori.

3. Evenly disperse 2 tablespoons of the sushi rice on top of the cream filling, covering it completely.

4. Place the carrots, the cucumbers, the bell peppers, and the snow pea shoots horizontally on top of the cream filling.

5. Begin to roll the sheet of nori from the bottom, over the vegetables, and then continue rolling until you have created a long tube. Cut the tube into 4 to 6 pieces of equal length.

6. Serve with the soy sauce or the Nama Shoyu for dipping.

DON'T LOSE YOUR TACOS

Raw, avocado-based

These simple tacos are great for kids and parties. Don't worry if you find yourself eating several of them. This is a high-vibration, quick-exit recipe!

MAKES 2 TO 4 SERVINGS

> **1 cup fresh Salsa Mole (page 220)**
>
> **4 large leaves cabbage or lettuce (or 4 sprouted-grain tortillas*)**

Place a dollop of the Salsa Mole inside the cabbage, lettuce leaves, or tortillas.

For you Texans out there—go ahead and shake on some Tabasco!

> *Note: You may use sprouted-grain tortillas instead of cabbage or lettuce leaves, but then this recipe would combine as a starch rather than as a raw food. Although sprouted-grain tortillas are not a "live" product, they are a great choice for this recipe. If you choose to adjust the recipe in this way, keep in mind that it will be considered a starch-based meal.*

DON'T LOSE YOUR CHEESY TACOS

Flesh category

When you taste the traditionally indulgent Italian flavors of the grated raw goat cheese, fresh tomato, and garlic you may momentarily forget that this is really a *live*, quick-exit recipe. It's delicious combinations like this one that make the Raw Food Life Force Energy diet so easy to love. Pile on the cheese, take a big bite, and let the juice dribble down your chin!

MAKES 2 SERVINGS

> ½ **cup chopped fresh cilantro**
>
> **1 cup diced tomato**
>
> **1 tablespoon minced fresh garlic**
>
> **Sea salt and fresh pepper to taste**
>
> **4 large leaves of cabbage or lettuce**
>
> **1 cup raw corn, cut off the cob**
>
> **1 cup shredded Alta Dena raw goat cheese**

Mix all of the ingredients, except the cabbage or lettuce leaves, in a mixing bowl. Toss and distribute the mixture onto the cabbage leaves. Pick one up with your hands and enjoy!

SWEET POTATO BEET PASTA WITH PESTO AND DICED TOMATOES

Neutral

I love the color and freshness of this dish. It makes a great alternative to a salad.

MAKES 2 SERVINGS

FOR THE PASTA:

1 medium sweet potato, peeled and either spiralized or cut into fine strips on the mandoline

1 large beet, peeled and either spiralized or cut into fine strips on the mandoline

FOR THE PESTO:

1 cup fresh basil

1 tablespoon cold-pressed, extra virgin olive oil

Sea salt and fresh pepper to taste

1 clove garlic, diced

1 medium tomato, diced

Place the sweet potato "pasta" and the beet "pasta" in two separate mounds on a plate. Setting aside the diced tomatoes, mix the pesto ingredients in a food processor until smooth. Place the pesto mixture on top of the mounds of pasta. Top with the diced tomatoes and enjoy!

RED BEET RAVIOLI STUFFED WITH TARRAGON GOAT CHEESE BY PURE FOOD AND WINE

This recipe comes straight from Pure Food and Wine, the legendary raw food restaurant in New York City. It is a must-dine venue for anyone who is interested in raw foods. Check out their website, www.purefoodandwine.com, and their packaged goods available online at www.oneluckyduck.com!

MAKES 6 TO 8 SERVINGS

> 3 cups pine nuts, soaked in water for 1 hour
>
> ¾ cups cold-pressed, extra virgin olive oil
>
> 2 whole lemons, peeled and quartered
>
> Zest of 2 lemons
>
> 1 medium shallot, minced
>
> 2 tablespoons nutritional yeast
>
> 2 teaspoons whole black peppercorns
>
> 1 clove garlic, minced
>
> Celtic sea salt and fresh ground pepper to taste
>
> ¾ cups roughly chopped tarragon, cleaned and stemmed
>
> 1 to 2 medium red beets, peeled and very thinly sliced

1. In a food processor, mix together the pine nuts, the olive oil, the lemons, and the zest for about 8 minutes. Pour half of this mixture into a blender and set the other half aside.

2. Add the yeast and 1 teaspoon of the peppercorns to the mixture in the blender and blend on medium speed for 2 minutes, until thick and smooth. This will be the "goat cheese." Transfer the blended mixture to a bowl and refrigerate, uncovered, for one hour.

3. Take the other half of the mixture that you set aside and place it in the blender. (This will be the sauce that will be placed under the ravioli.)

4. Add the remaining peppercorns to this mixture along with the garlic, shallots, and ¾ cups of water.

5. Blend on high for 1 minute, until it achieves a smooth, runny consistency, then salt to taste.

6. Once the "goat cheese" from step 2 has completely cooled, fold ½ cup of the tarragon into it, then salt to taste.

7. Spoon about 1 tablespoon of the cheese onto each of the beet slices, then top these with the remaining beet slices.

8. To serve, pour the sauce from step 5 onto a deep serving platter and place the ravioli on top. Sprinkle with the remaining tarragon, and add salt and pepper to taste.

RAW TERIYAKI "STIR-FRY"

Neutral

MAKES 2 SERVINGS

2 medium carrots, julienned

2 medium portobello mushrooms, sliced

¼ cup diced sweet onions

1 medium red bell pepper, julienned

¼ cup soy sauce or Nama Shoyu

¼ cup pure grade B maple syrup

1 tablespoon diced fresh ginger

1 tablespoon diced fresh garlic

1 cup "sushi rice" (page 188)

In a mixing bowl, mix all of the ingredients together and let marinate for at least 2 hours before serving, or let the mixture marinate for up to 48 hours for maximum flavor. Serve over the "sushi rice."

QUICKEST SPAGHETTI

Neutral.*

MAKES 2 SERVINGS

> **2 large zucchinis, sliced into pasta-like strips with a mandoline or a spiralizer**
>
> **½ cup Seeds of Change pasta sauce (see note)**
>
> **½ cup grated raw Alta Dena goat cheese (optional*)**

In a small sauce pan, heat the pasta sauce well and pour over the zucchini. Toss and top with the goat cheese if desired.

> *Note: This brand of pasta sauce is the best tasting and healthiest bottled sauce I have found so far, and it is easy to find in the local health food store. Other organic, high-quality pasta sauces are acceptable too, but look for little to no sugars (never refined sugars), and oil (only olive oil) listed as one of the last ingredients.*

> **If you add the goat cheese, this dish will no longer be neutral; it will combine as a "flesh" dish.*

SANDWICHES

These sandwiches are so quick and easy to make, you can enjoy them at any time, and they are great for transporting—whether for flights, school lunches, or picnics. Pair them with some raw vegetables or a salad, and you will have a delicious, satisfying meal!

Some of the sandwiches call for a specialty raw bread product made by the raw food bakery Good Stuff. You can order these breads online at www.live-live.com. Made of vegetables and seeds, they come in the form of adorable miniature loaves and are convenient for anyone who loves bread but is trying to avoid grain.

RAW OPEN-FACED SANDWICHES

Raw, nut-based

MAKES 6 OPEN-FACED SANDWICHES

> **6 slices Good Stuff "Raw Rye" or "Down Home Harvest" bread
> (the equivalent of about half a miniature loaf)**
>
> **2 tablespoons Dijon mustard**
>
> **1 large tomato, sliced**
>
> **½ cup alfalfa sprouts**

Lay the bread slices on a flat surface or cutting board. Spread on the mustard, then add the tomato slices and the alfalfa sprouts.

NUT-BUTTER AND JELLY SANDWICHES

Raw, nut-based

MAKES 2 MINI-SANDWICHES

> **4 slices Good Stuff "Raw Rye" or "Down Home Harvest" bread**
>
> **3 tablespoons raw almond butter**
>
> **3 tablespoons 100 percent pure fruit jam of your choice
> (I recommend the Sorrell Ridge or St. Dalfour brand)**

Lay the bread slices on a flat surface or cutting board. Spread on the almond butter, then layer the jam on top. Enjoy the sandwiches open- or close-faced.

PORTOBELLO-MARINARA GRANDWICH

Starch

When you have a hearty appetite, this is a wonderfully "meaty," satisfying sandwich!

MAKES 2 OPEN-FACED SANDWICHES

> 2 portobello mushrooms, stemmed and sliced
>
> Sea salt and fresh pepper to taste
>
> 2 slices sprouted-grain bread
>
> ¼ cup Seeds of Change tomato-basil pasta sauce, heated
>
> 1 avocado, sliced
>
> 1 beefsteak tomato, sliced
>
> 1 sweet onion, sliced
>
> 6 leaves arugula
>
> 4 leaves fresh basil
>
> 1 tablespoon chopped oregano

1. Heat ¼ cup of water in a frying pan and add the mushrooms with the salt and pepper sprinkled on top.

2. Cook the mushrooms on high heat until they are juicy throughout (about 5 minutes).

3. Lay the bread slices on a cutting board. Spread on the pasta sauce, then place 3 or 4 mushroom slices on each slice (enough to cover the bread). Layer on the avocado, the tomato, the onion, the arugula, the basil, and finally the oregano. Since this sandwich can be messy to eat with your hands, you may prefer to eat it close-faced or with a fork and knife.

AVOCADO WRAP

Starch

MAKES 4 BABY WRAPS

> 4 large leaves purple or white cabbage
>
> 2 tablespoons Dijon mustard
>
> 1 medium, ripe avocado
>
> 1 medium tomato, chopped
>
> ¼ cup chopped cilantro

Place all ingredients inside the cabbage leaves, distributing evenly, and enjoy!

SALAD SANDWICH

Starch

MAKES 2 OPEN-FACED SANDWICHES

¼ cup alfalfa sprouts

1 red or orange bell pepper, julienned

¼ medium cucumber, thinly sliced

½ avocado, sliced

1 tablespoon finely chopped parsley

1 tablespoon finely chopped cilantro

1 tablespoon Dijon mustard

Spike, all-purpose herbal seasoning, to taste

4 slices sprouted-grain bread

Mix all of the ingredients except the bread in a mixing bowl and then distribute the mixture evenly between the bread slices to make two open-faced sandwiches. Whatever is left over may be enjoyed as a side salad.

COOKED VEGETARIAN ENTRÉES

I like to think of these recipes as "the new comfort food." We turn to these dishes when we want cozy, warm, hearty dishes that offer all the comforts of familiar flavors and fullness but with none of the drawbacks.

Keep in mind that while these dishes are not actually raw, they are extremely helpful for transitioning off of mainstream and common vegetarian fare. Adhering to the "light-to-heavy" principle, I recommend serving these and other cooked entrées mainly as dinner dishes. However, even the grain-based starch dishes are made mostly of vegetables, so they are still very high up on the list of cleansing, energizing dishes.

PARSNIP-CARROT-BEET BAKE

Neutral

MAKES 2 TO 4 SERVINGS

2 large parsnips, sliced into thin disks

3 large carrots, sliced into thin disks

1 large beet (or 2 to 3 small ones), sliced into thin disks

3 tablespoons agave nectar

Sea salt and fresh pepper to taste

Preheat oven to 350° F. In a baking dish, layer the parsnips, carrots, and beets. In a small bowl, mix the agave with the salt and pepper, then pour the agave mixture evenly over the vegetables. Bake until the veggies become tender, brown, and crispy on the edges (about 25 minutes). Serve on a platter, family-style.

PORTOBELLO MELTS

Flesh category

MAKES 2 SERVINGS

> **2 portobello mushrooms, stemmed and left whole**
>
> **Sea salt and pepper to taste**
>
> **½ cup Seeds of Change tomato-basil pasta sauce, heated**
>
> **4 ounces raw cheddar-style goat cheese (I recommend the Alta Dena brand), grated**
>
> **¼ cup chopped fresh basil or oregano (optional)**

Heat ¼ cup of water in a frying pan and add the portobello mushrooms with the salt and pepper sprinkled on top. Cook the mushrooms on high heat until they are juicy throughout (about 5 minutes). Place them on a plate and cover them with the pasta sauce and the grated cheese. Top with the fresh basil or oregano.

PORTOBELLO STEAKS AND BURGERS

Starch

MAKES 2 BURGERS

4 portobello mushrooms, stemmed and left whole

¼ cup or Nama Shoyu or regular soy sauce

¼ cup pure grade B maple syrup

2 sprouted-grain burger buns (I recommend the Alverado St. Bakery brand)

2 beefsteak (or any large) tomatoes, sliced

4 leaves organic lettuce

1 large sweet onion, sliced

4 tablespoons Dijon mustard (Westbrae is my favorite brand and is available at most health food stores) and/or natural ketchup (I like the one by Annie's) and/or A1 steak sauce

In a bowl, mix the Nama Shoyu and the maple syrup. Place the portobellos in the mixture and let soak for at least 1 hour. Preheat oven to 350° F. In a baking dish, place the portobellos in the oven and bake for about 20 minutes, or until they start to look plump and juicy. Toast the buns. Place two portobellos on each, then layer on the vegetables and the condiments. Serve like a regular burger.

AGE OF AQUARIUS MAC 'N' CHEESE

Starch with some flesh*

MAKES 2 SERVINGS

> 2 cups spelt or Kamut or brown rice pasta elbows, uncooked (any brand will do)
>
> 1 tablespoon organic butter
>
> 3 ounces raw cheddar-style goat cheese, grated
>
> Sea salt and fresh pepper to taste

Cook the pasta elbows in boiling water until soft (about 8 minutes) and then rinse well. In a saucepan, heat the pasta with the butter and the cheese, covered on low until the cheese is fully melted (about 2 minutes). Add the sea salt and the pepper and serve while hot!

> *This recipe is not an ideal combination because it mixes starch with cheese (flesh). However, it is a great choice of comfort food for children or friends who are interested in trying out this diet.*

SWEET BUTTERNUT HEAVEN

Starch

MAKES 2 SERVINGS

> 3 cups cubed butternut squash
>
> ¼ cup pure maple syrup
>
> 2 teaspoons pumpkin pie spice
>
> 2 teaspoons organic butter
>
> Sea salt to taste

Preheat oven to 350° F. In a mixing bowl, mix all of the ingredients well and then place them evenly distributed in a baking dish. Bake uncovered for about 35 minutes or until they are soft and brown on the edges.

MEGA-VEGGIE PLATTER

Neutral

MAKES 2 GENEROUS SERVINGS

> 15 to 20 spears fresh asparagus, steamed
>
> 2 cups diced fresh tomatoes
>
> 2 cups steamed bok choy
>
> 2 cups fresh raw corn cut off the cob
>
> 2 tablespoons, cold-pressed, extra virgin olive oil
>
> 3 tablespoons balsamic vinegar
>
> Sea salt and fresh pepper to taste

On a large square or rectangular serving platter, stack the vegetables on top of each other, in the above order. Dress with olive oil, balsamic vinegar, the salt and pepper to taste.

SWEET BASIL TOMATO TOWERS

Flesh category

MAKES 2 SERVINGS

2 medium tomatoes, sliced

10 fresh basil leaves

1 small sweet onion, sliced

1 tablespoon cold-pressed, extra virgin olive oil

1 tablespoon balsamic vinegar

Sea salt and fresh pepper to taste

3 ounces raw goat cheese (if hard, shredded; if soft, it will be spread)

In a mixing bowl, gently toss the tomatoes, basil, and onion, and fully coat them with the olive oil, vinegar, and salt and pepper. Next, build two towers starting with a base of tomatoes, followed by goat cheese, basil, and onion. If there is any remaining dressing in the bowl, drizzle it artfully around the towers and serve!

Tip: To avoid toppling a whole tower with the first slice, use a very sharp knife that will easily cut through the vegetables when eating this.

KOMBU MELT

Flesh category

MAKES 2 SERVINGS

> 3 packages soft Kombu (seaweed) noodles, rinsed
>
> 1 head broccoli, cut into florets
>
> 1 cup shiitake mushrooms, whole or sliced
>
> 1 to 1 ½ cups Seeds of Change marinara sauce
>
> 4 ounces raw cheddar-style goat cheese (I recommend the Alta Dena brand), grated

1. Preheat oven to 250° F. On the stovetop, steam the broccoli in a steamer and heat the pasta sauce in a saucepan.

2. When the broccoli is nearly soft, place the noodles in the steamer (with the broccoli) just long enough to heat them (about 1 minute). The noodles need only be warmed, not cooked, as they are already soft.

3. Place the noodles either in an ovenproof plate or in a baking dish, topped with the broccoli florets, mushrooms, and the heated marinara sauce. Finally, sprinkle with cheese and place the whole dish in the oven at 250° F with the door ajar for 3 minutes, or until the cheese has melted.

NO-FRY STIR-FRY

Neutral

MAKES 2 TO 4 SERVINGS

½ cup vegetable broth (optional; water may be used instead)

1 teaspoon organic butter

1 cup cauliflower florets

1 cup broccoli florets

½ cup sliced shiitake mushrooms

½ cup julienned carrots

½ cup snow peas

½ cup baby corn cut off the cob (optional)

1 cup mung bean sprouts

¼ cup chopped fresh cilantro

¼ cup chopped fresh basil

1 tablespoon chopped fresh mint (optional)

1 tablespoon diced garlic

1 tablespoon diced fresh ginger

1 cup Nama Shoyu

1 cup pure Grade B maple syrup

Heat a wok or a skillet on high heat with ½ cup of water or vegetable broth and the organic butter. In a large mixing bowl, toss all of the vegetables, except the mung sprouts and the herbs. Place this mixture in the wok and cook on medium heat for about 5 minutes or until just tender. Plate the heated mixture over the mung sprouts and top with the herbs. Enjoy!

SEAFOOD ENTRÉES

Seafood is really helpful when you are transitioning to the Raw Food Life Force Energy lifestyle and aren't ready to eat all raw or vegetarian while cleansing. Obviously, if you are interested only in all raw and/or vegetarian recipes, you should skip this section.

The great thing about fresh fish (preferably wild) is that it is really easy to digest. Therefore, these recipes offer all of the gourmet appeal of great seafood without interfering with body cleansing. Although I do use small amounts of butter for pan searing and baking, I make sure it's organic butter, which is the best fat to cook with—and as long it's used in small amounts, it will not weigh the body down. So, ahoy and enjoy!

BEET THIS FLOUNDER!

Flesh

MAKES 2 SERVINGS

2 half-pound flounder or trout filets, rinsed

1 cup chopped beets

1 clove garlic, diced

2 tablespoons fresh-squeezed lemon juice

1 teaspoon organic butter, melted

Sea salt and fresh pepper to taste

1 cup raw corn cut off the cob

2 to 4 sprigs of your favorite herb, such as chives, parsley, or sage (optional)

Preheat oven to 450° F. Place the fish filets in a shallow baking dish, then add the beets, and then distribute the garlic, lemon juice, butter, and salt and pepper evenly over the whole dish. Bake covered for 25 minutes or until the fish begins to flake. On two separate plates, place ½ cup of the raw corn and top with the baked fish and beets. Garnish each plate with a sprig or two of your favorite herb to add color and a festive spirit!

SIMPLE SPIKED SNAPPER

Flesh

MAKES 2 SERVINGS

> 2 half-pound red snapper filets, rinsed
>
> 2 tablespoons fresh-squeezed lemon juice
>
> 1 tablespoon organic butter
>
> 1 clove garlic, diced
>
> Spike seasoning to taste

Preheat oven to 450° F. Place the fish in a baking dish, add the lemon juice, dab the filets with butter, add the garlic, and sprinkle on the Spike seasoning to taste. Bake covered for approximately 25 minutes or until the fish begins to flake.

HAS-TO-BE HALIBUT

Flesh

MAKES 2 SERVINGS

> 2 half-pound fresh halibut filets, rinsed
>
> ¼ cup white wine
>
> 1 teaspoon organic butter
>
> 2 tablespoons agave nectar
>
> Sea salt and fresh pepper to taste

Preheat oven to 450° F. Place the fish in a baking dish, add the white wine, dab the filets with butter, and add the agave nectar and the salt and pepper. Bake covered for approximately 25 minutes or until the fish begins to flake and sizzle.

HERB-ENCRUSTED SWORDFISH

Flesh

MAKES 2 SERVINGS

1 teaspoon organic butter, melted

1 clove garlic, diced

1 tablespoon finely chopped sage

1 tablespoon finely chopped rosemary

1 tablespoon finely chopped chives

1 tablespoon finely chopped thyme

Sea salt and fresh pepper to taste

2 half-pound swordfish filets, rinsed

Preheat oven to 450° F. In a bowl, mix the melted butter with the garlic, herbs, salt, and pepper. Coat the fish filets with the mixture by dipping them into the bowl.

Place the fish filets in a baking dish, and top with the remaining butter-garlic-herb mixture. Bake covered for approximately 25 minutes or until the fish is cooked through to taste (some people like their swordfish medium rare, whereas others like it cooked all the way through).

BREAKFAST ANY OTHER TIME

As you've learned, fresh fruits and juices of fruits and vegetables are the only ideal substances to consume before lunchtime. But where does that leave our beloved omelets, pancakes, and bagels? The good news is that you can still enjoy them—just avoid having them in the morning hours, and make them with the highest-quality ingredients and in the best combinations. Lunch and dinner are the perfect times to have these old favorites.

If you replace regular white bagels and flour with sprouted-grain bagels and the highest-quality whole-grain flours, you can indulge in your favorite breakfast-style foods while remaining well within the parameters of the Raw Food Life Force Energy diet. So wake up and smell the green juice, and look forward to having breakfast for lunch!

For you hard-core raw food devotees, check out the totally raw, nut-based pancakes and granola. There's truly something for everyone here.

THE GREAT PANCAKE AWAKENING

Starch*

No one should have to give up the joy of pancakes. In fact, I loved the fluffy, bready stuff drenched in maple syrup so much that I became a bit of a pancake connoisseur for some time. Granted, pancakes are not the ideal food to consume on a daily basis, but these pancakes are perfectly safe for the occasional indulgence. Stack 'em up and wash 'em down with some nice Chai-spiked almond milk!

MAKES ABOUT 6 PANCAKES

> **1 cup spelt or Kamut flour**
>
> **1 organic egg (optional*)**
>
> **1 cup Pacific or fresh almond milk**
>
> **Cinnamon, nutmeg, and ground clove to taste**
>
> **2 drops vanilla extract**
>
> **½ tablespoon organic butter**
>
> **¼ cup pure maple syrup**

In a mixing bowl, thoroughly whisk together all of the ingredients (except the maple syrup and butter) until you have a perfectly smooth batter. Heat the butter in a skillet at high heat. Using about ½ cup at a time, place medium-sized disks of pancake batter in the skillet and cook for about 3 minutes on each side. Top with the maple syrup. Delicious!

> *Tip: If you serve the pancakes on a dark-colored plate, you can sprinkle on a little Stevia around the dish to create the look of powdered sugar.*

> **The egg in this recipe prevents it from being perfectly combined, but since only one egg is being used for about 6 pancakes, it is not worth worrying about.*

REALLY RAW PANCAKES

Raw, nut-based*

I love these pancakes. Sometimes I eat them as part of a raw meal with or after a raw salad!

MAKES 1 TO 2 SERVINGS

> **1 to 3 raw pancakes by The Raw Bakery (sold in packs of 3 online at www.therawbakery.com)**
>
> **1 cup sliced banana**
>
> **¼ cup pure maple syrup**

Top the pancakes with banana and maple syrup, and dig in!

> *The raw pancakes are made of dates and flax seeds, so they combine as a nut-based meal.*

FRITTATA AL FRESCO

Flesh

Although eggs may not be an *ideal* food, they are ideal for transitioning into the Raw Food Life Force Energy diet because they are a very quick-exit flesh protein, which people need as they begin to break away from their old eating patterns. When eggs are well combined, as in this recipe, they won't weigh you down.

MAKES 1 SERVING

> **4 organic eggs**
>
> **1 to 2 ounces raw goat cheese**
>
> **¼ cup diced tomatoes**
>
> **1 teaspoon organic butter**
>
> **1 tablespoon chopped rosemary or thyme**

Preheat oven to 350° F. Whisk the eggs thoroughly in a bowl. Heat the butter in a skillet at high heat and add the eggs, then top with the goat cheese and the herbs. Bake covered in the skillet for 10 minutes or until plump and firm. Serve with garden greens.

BAGELS AND "GREEN" CHEESE

Starch

Okay, so it's not exactly cream cheese, but it's creamy, delicious, and good for you to boot. Another idea is simply to toast the bagel with a touch of butter and raw honey, which my kids love.

MAKES 1 SERVING

> **2 avocado slices**
>
> **1 sprouted-grain bagel, sliced in half**
>
> **Pinch sea salt**
>
> **1 teaspoon agave nectar (optional)**

Spread the avocado on the bagel. Sprinkle on the sea salt and drizzle on the agave nectar if desired. This bagel is delicious toasted or untoasted.

THE BEST THING SINCE SLICED BREAD

Starch

This is really simple but so delicious. Enjoy it with a big salad for a simple lunch or dinner. Some of my clients like to have this for dessert after a starch/salad meal.

MAKES 1 TO 2 SERVINGS

> **2 slices sprouted-grain bread**
>
> **1 teaspoon organic butter**
>
> **1 to 2 teaspoons raw honey**

Toast the bread, then spread on the butter and the honey!

RAW GRANOLA

Raw, nut-based

All of you granola lovers out there, take note: all mainstream granolas are cooked in oils and combine starch (oats) with seeds and nuts, creating a very heavy, hard-to-digest combination. This recipe, made with Lydia's wonderful Grainless Apple Granola, which you can order online from www.therawfooddetoxdiet.com or in the raw food section of your local health food store, is the solution to your granola cravings. It is made of nuts, seeds, and dried fruits. Enjoy it alone as a snack, with a salad, or as a raw dessert.

MAKES 1 SERVING

¼ cup Lydia's Grainless Apple Granola

1 medium banana, sliced

¼ cup Pacific or fresh almond milk

1 tablespoon agave nectar or 1 packet Stevia

Mix all of the ingredients together in a cereal bowl and grab the nearest spoon!

SIDES AND SNACKS

SALSA MOLE

Avocado-based

MAKES 2½ CUPS

1 cup chopped Roma or Holland tomatoes

2 ripe avocados, diced

¼ to ½ cup chopped fresh cilantro

1 tablespoon diced garlic

¼ cup fresh-squeezed lime juice

3 tablespoons agave nectar

Sea salt and fresh ground pepper to taste

½ cup fresh corn cut off the cob

In a medium-sized bowl, mix together all of the ingredients well or until creamy as desired. Try Salsa Mole in any number of ways: serve it with raw veggies, use it to create a sprouted-grain tortilla wrap, place a dollop on a slice of sprouted-grain toast, or serve it on top of a plate of greens to create a rich avocado salad.

VEGGIE CHIPS AND DIP

Avocado-based

MAKES 3 CUPS OF VEGETABLE "CHIPS" AND 2½ CUPS OF DIP

1 cup thinly sliced carrots

1 cup thinly sliced parsnips

1 cup thinly sliced sweet potato or jicama (Mexican potato: jicama are hydrating and crunchy like an apple but not sweet)

1 cup Salsa Mole (page 216)

Artfully arrange each type of "chip" on a plate with the Salsa Mole in the middle for a colorful snack. Grab a chip and dig for Salsa Mole!

DESSERTS

The following desserts are actually beautifying, slimming treats. I indulge in one of these desserts on a daily basis and highly recommend them to anyone who loves sweets but wants to maintain, or boost their levels of Life Force Energy. Since most of these desserts are based on tree fruits and nuts (such as dried fruits, avocados, and coconuts), they are among the highest–Life Force Energy recipes in this book, second only to the all-raw salad recipes. Now you have every reason to indulge that sweet tooth.

MILK THAT SHAKES & SHAPES

Combines with a raw, avocado-based meal or a raw, nut-based meal

MAKES 3 CUPS

 1 cup Pacific almond milk

 1 medium organic banana

 2 to 4 tablespoons pure cocoa powder

 4 fresh medjool dates, pitted

 ½ cup crushed ice or 4 to 6 ice cubes

Blend all ingredients in a high-powered blender and enjoy as a dessert or a snack.

CHOCOLATE MOUSSE

Combines with a raw, avocado-based meal and a raw, nut-based meal, or after a fresh fruit meal.

MAKES 1 TO 2 SERVINGS

 2 young coconuts, meat scooped out

 3 heaping tablespoons pure cocoa powder

 5 fresh medjool dates, pitted

In a food processor, combine the ingredients and blend until smooth. I recommend serving the mousse in a chilled short glass or a small glass bowl.

ALL-PURPOSE RAW VANILLA CASHEW CREAM BY IBRAHIM "IBO" GENCAY OF THE RAW BAKERY

Raw, nut-based

Ibo Gencay is the executive chef and CEO of The Raw Bakery, a leading raw food company, which produces some of the best premade raw food items available. I highly recommend checking out The Raw Bakery goods, particularly their brownies and macaroons! You can order them from the company's website at www.therawbakery.com or by calling 1-800-571-8369.

MAKES 4 CUPS

3½ cups cashew nuts (soaked for 4 to 8 hours)

½ cup raw honey

1 teaspoon vanilla extract or the seeds of 1 vanilla bean

1 teaspoon extra virgin raw coconut oil

Place all of the ingredients and ¼ to ½ cup of water (to facilitate blending) in a food processor and and blend well until smooth. Refrigerate for at least 1 hour and serve chilled.

BANANA MINT

Combines with a raw, avocado-based meal and a raw, nut-based meal, or after a fresh fruit meal.

Mint lovers will dreamily scoop up this creamy, cold mint ice cream!

MAKES 2 SERVINGS

> **3 medium or large frozen bananas, cut in thirds**
>
> **1 teaspoon chopped fresh, mint leaves**
>
> **Organic chocolate chips (optional)**

In a food processor, mix the bananas and the mint together and serve. Top with or mix in your favorite organic chocolate chips for a "mint-chip" version!

LEMON MERINGUE MOUSSE

Raw, avocado-based

MAKES ABOUT 1½ CUPS

> **1 avocado, pitted and scooped out of the skin**
>
> **3 or 4 fresh medjool dates, pitted and soaked**
>
> **½ tablespoon maple syrup**
>
> **½ lemon with peel**
>
> **2 tablespoons chopped nuts of your choice (optional)**

In a food processor, thoroughly blend together all of the ingredients except the nuts until smooth. Garnish with a thin half slice of fresh lemon and a sprinkling of your favorite chopped nuts, if desired.

"BAKED" APPLES

Fresh fruit category

MAKES 2 TO 4 SERVINGS

> 2 fuji apples, sliced very thinly (tip: use a mandoline)
>
> ¼ teaspoon ground cinnamon
>
> ¼ teaspoon ground nutmeg
>
> ¼ teaspoon ground clove
>
> 2 tablespoons pure maple syrup
>
> 1 teaspoon vanilla extract
>
> A dollop All-Purpose Raw Vanilla Cashew Cream (optional; see page 224)

In a baking dish, spread out the apple slices. In a small bowl, whisk together all of the other ingredients. Pour the mixture on top of the apples. Top with All-Purpose Raw Vanilla Cashew Cream, if desired. Enjoy right away or keep refrigerated until ready to serve. The longer the apples sit in the liquid mixture, the more flavorful the dish becomes.

BANANA CREAM SUPREME ICE CREAM

Combines with a raw, avocado-based meal and a raw, nut-based meal, or after a fresh fruit meal.

This is a remarkably creamy ice cream. I love it for dessert after an all-fruit meal or an avocado salad.

MAKES 2 TO 3 CUPS

> **3 frozen bananas, cut into thirds**
>
> **6 medjool dates**
>
> **1 tablespoon pure maple syrup and/or pure cocoa powder (optional)**

In a high-speed blender, place the dates and several pieces of the frozen banana along with a splash of water. Blend on high and then add the rest of the bananas and blend well until creamy. Top with the pure maple syrup and/or the pure cocoa powder, if desired.

CHERRY CHOCOLATE DREAM

Fresh fruit category

This simple dish is great for entertaining.

MAKES 2 SERVINGS

>   **1 cup pure maple syrup**
>
>   **3 heaping tablespoons pure cocoa powder**
>
>   **1 cup fresh cherries**
>
>   **Fresh strawberry and banana wedges (optional)**

To make the chocolate sauce, in a blender, blend the cocoa powder and the syrup until uniform. Place the cherries on a plate next to a bowl of the chocolate sauce. Dip and dream! Add strawberries and banana wedges for variety and extra color.

FREQUENTLY ASKED QUESTIONS

So many people have similar questions as they undertake this diet lifestyle that I'd like to take this opportunity to address the most commonly asked questions. If you have a question that is not answered here or in one of my books, feel free to send an e-mail to natalia@therawfooddetoxdiet.com. I love reading your e-mails and hearing your questions. Your personal success stories always move and inspire me.

Can I make the vegetable juice elixirs the night before and store them for the next day?

While the Life Force Energy of the juice peaks the moment it is prepared and the in-tegrity of the enzymes is compromised when exposed to air (oxidation), you will still benefit tremendously from drinking the juice even hours after making it if you keep it very cold in an air-tight container. By the time you drink it, the juice will still be chock-full of precious chlorophyll, organic hydration, minerals, and many vitamins and enzymes.

Remember that while I recommend drinking the juice first thing every day, you will benefit from drinking it at any time during the day as long as it is on an empty stomach. Therefore, if it suits your schedule better, you could also enjoy it several hours after your lunch meal or an hour before dinner. Many of my clients make a large amount of juice in the late afternoon or evening, drinking some right away and then freezing the remainder for the next morning. When I travel, I always freeze some that I can defrost and enjoy the next day. I know that it is still full of Life Force Energy because both my body and my mind are awakened immediately upon drinking it!

Is there a way to continue having my coffee in the morning around the fruit and vegetable juice until I'm ready to give it up?

Until you make the decision to give up coffee, feel free to enjoy coffee at least thirty minutes before or after drinking the fruit and vegetable juice. Eventually, when you discover that the elixirs charge you up more than the coffee, you'll surely nix the coffee. But there's no need to rush the transition away from coffee—it is a far lesser evil than the dense foods and slow-exit combinations.

How long should I wait to eat after a vegetable juice?

Ten to fifteen minutes is usually long enough for eight to thirty ounces. But if you drink more than thirty ounces, I recommend waiting at least forty-five minutes.

I'm traveling to Europe this summer. How can I enjoy the food there without compromising my diet?

Mediterranean destinations such as Italy, France, Spain, and Greece are easy places to incorporate the program. You'll have access to abundant fresh fruit and avocados for salads. In restaurants you can order plates of steamed veggies with sides of marinara sauce and goat cheese (don't worry if it's not raw) to eat with your salads for lunch, and you can order amazing fresh fish, salads, veggies, and wine for dinner. Take your 70 percent (+) chocolate bars for dessert and you'll be all set.

What do you do about the vegetable juice when you travel? Is there any way to substitute it?

I don't expect to find the green juice when I travel and I am not the kind of person to travel with a juicer (though some of my clients do). If I'm going somewhere within the United States I'm usually able to find at least one juice bar in the area posted on-line. When I travel abroad and cannot locate a juice bar, I just do without. It's not ideal, but when you drink vegetable juice all year round you can afford to miss a week! Having said that, I do take enough frozen Life Force Power-ade (page 158) to see me through the flight, protect against jet lag, and keep my immunity boosted.

When you can't get fresh vegetable juice, just be vigilant about getting as much Life Force Energy from your meals and environment as possible. An ideal daily in-take scenario "on the raw energy road" looks something like this: when you're hungry enjoy fresh fruit as desired with herbal tea, lemon, and Stevia (optional). Lunch can consist of fruit and then a large raw veggie salad with avocado, dates, and bananas or some steamed veggies. Dinner could be a raw salad, steamed veggies, and fish (vegetarians can enjoy a steamed or grilled veggie plate) with the dark chocolate for dessert. I always take plenty of Green & Black or Dagoba chocolate bars with me.

One of my big travel secrets is not to consume anything on the plane other than vegetable juice. I don't expect many of you to be ready to do that (though it makes a huge difference to your digestion and jet lag and pays off over the following days). If you do eat on board, eat only what you bring with you and choose among the most hydrating foods (fruits, veggies, maybe a veggie sandwich or a salad with a Lara bar or other raw treat). It also helps to eat as close to the end of the flight as possible since your digestion slows down dramatically when you're in transit. Couple slow digestion with dehydration and you can see why flying is so constipating!

Does everything have to be organic?

In the beginning, the most important thing to do is get used to the new foods and quick-exit combinations. If you find it too stressful, don't worry about whether your food is organic. Eventually, once you have your bearings and you are shopping at high-quality grocery stores, you will find it's actually quite easy and not much more expensive to buy organic produce.

Besides, in my experience, the typical person starting out on this lifestyle is far too impacted with old waste matter and out of harmony with his/her natural vibrations to pick up on the subtle harmonic differences of organic produce anyway. Eventually, as your body gets cleaner and more rightly vibing, you will naturally gravitate toward the organic produce. Even then, you may find (as I do) that some nonorganic produce items still make their way into your kitchen.

There are some things I will buy only organic: greens, all vegetables for juicing, bananas, and avocados. There are many things—such as raw corn, navel oranges, winter grapefruit, and watermelon—that just don't look or taste as good from the organic departments. Since I really enjoy these items, I buy and eat the ones that look and taste the best without worrying about the fact that they are not organic. What's important is the big picture of your food intake, so don't obsess over the organic issue. You'll get there when you get there, and in the meantime you can be raising your vibrations and cleansing deeply by just applying the Raw Food Energy principles outlined in Part I of this book.

Can you eat neutral foods anytime?

Neutral foods such as raw veggies and dark chocolate may be enjoyed anytime, but try to avoid constant eating as it inhibits digestive rest, which is a key to renewing the body.

How does young coconut meat combine?

Young coconut meat combines with veggies, starches, and nuts/seeds/dried fruit, but don't mix it with flesh or cheese. (The *water* from the young coconuts is neutral, so you can combine that with anything.)

When can I have raw treats such as the raw flaxseed crackers, raw brownies, Larabars, etc.? Can I enjoy them after an avocado salad? What about after fish?

You will find all you need to know about how to combine foods by reading the ingredients. If it is made of raw nuts and/or dried fruit, you'll know that the food will combine with anything else in that category. The raw treats are just nut/seed/dried fruit concoctions, so simply combine them with that category of foods. I recommend eating them as part of a meal rather than in between meals to avoid taking dense food in at every interval. For example, enjoy them with a big raw salad for lunch. Since they are nut-based, they do not go with avocados or fish. However, The Raw Bakery has created "nutless macaroons" that go perfectly with avocados. Check them out at www.therawbakery.com.

I'm confused about how avocados combine. Can you explain?

Avocados typically combine as a starch, meaning they will go with breads, grains, cooked root vegetables, and legumes but not with flesh/cheese or any other categories. *However*, they are one of the odd exceptions because they *do* combine with fresh and dried fruits (avocados are technically a fruit themselves), yet they do *not* combine with nuts. Bananas are also an exception as they combine with fresh fruits and dried fruits. This means that you can have bananas as a "dessert" after an avocado and raw veggie salad!

Are there any times when fruit will combine with other foods?

Fruits do mix with green veggies and they may even be blended with greens in green vegetable juices or in a raw soup. Also, if you're eating an entirely raw meal (such as a raw vegetable soup and avocado salad), you can enjoy a recipe that calls for a small amount of fresh fruit (such as a raw strawberry ice cream or the "Baked" Apples (page 226). Technically, it is not a perfect combination, but in the first few years of eating this way, your body won't be sensitive enough to react too much to it. What matters most is that you do what works best for you. Just be sure that you don't incorporate any cooked food if you're going to have fruit.

Is "raw bread" a sprouted-grain bread like Ezekiel? If not, where do I find it? And what makes a "raw bread" raw?

The Ezekiel and Alverado St. Bakery breads are *not* raw because they are heated above 118° F, but they are very easily digested, which makes them a quick-exit bread and very useful in transition stages.

The best totally raw breads I've ever tasted are made by a company called The Good Stuff by Mom & Me. You can find their products online at *www.gimmegoodstuff .com* or call 888-797-6865. They have great raw mini-loaves that I love to top with raw honey and/or raw almond butter, pesto or mustard, sprouts, and tomatoes for open-faced sandwiches!

A lot of raw foodists use psyllium, should I try it?

Personally, I *do not* recommend using psyllium unless you are doing it in conjunction with colonics. Psyllium expands ten times its weight in the body, which, if your body does not expel all that it draws up, could turn into a very uncomfortable if not dangerous experience. Psyllium and bentonite clay together will draw up postputrefactive matter, which is wonderful to eliminate, but unless you are prepared to do several colonics to ensure the passage of this extremely dense waste matter, I do not recommend it.

What is a good snack when you're hungry but running out the door?

Veggies are always safe since you don't have to worry about your combos. But your ideal snack choice really depends on when you're having it and how long after a meal, and whether you want something in a different food group from what you ate previously. For example, if you are snacking within the same food group as your latest meal, you can safely snack on anything from that same category. But if you are switching categories, you must wait at least three hours between them. I don't recommend much snacking, but I know most people want something between about 3 and 5 P.M.

If you are going to snack, try to make it raw, as the best snacks are hydrating and enzyme rich, such as raw veggies or veggie juice. Fruits can be good if you have them at least three to four hours after lunch. The raw cheeses are great to have before a flesh/vegetable combo dinner. (I often enjoy some Alta Dena raw cheese before going out.)

I really like hummus. How does it fit into this diet?

Traditional hummus can be combined as a starch. However, because it is made up of chickpeas, which are difficult to digest, and includes tahini (sesame seeds and chickpeas, a legume/starch and a poor combo), I do not recommended it for anyone who is trying to lose weight. If you really love hummus, keep it simple—enjoy it just with veggies and never with flesh or nuts. If you are just starting out on this diet, then it shouldn't hold you back; but as you progress you will find it doesn't increase energy or encourage weight loss.

There are some good raw hummus recipes out there. Try the one from *Raw Food, Real World* by Matthew Kenney and Sarma Melngailis, New York: Regan, 2005. Raw hummus is typically made of nuts instead of chickpeas, so combine accordingly.

How much wine can I have and when?

Wine is neutral in terms of food combining, and a little bit now and then will not hold you back. Surprisingly, it does not appear to interfere with my clients' weight loss efforts. However, it will affect your *energy* level. So, feel free to have some wine with dinner when you desire it. It is a much lesser evil than white flour, processed foods, and refined sugar, but keep in mind that any alcoholic beverage will disrupt the harmony of your vibrations, reduce your energy, and act as a depressant. Since wine is a liquid, it will not weigh down the system. So, overall: doable but certainly not Life Force Energy generating.

I want to maintain my muscle mass. Where do I get my protein?

Leafy greens, green vegetable juice (as in the Life Force Power-ade), sea vegetables, raw nuts and nut butters, and raw goat cheese are all rich in protein. You can still eat flesh products as desired in this diet lifestyle as long as they are well combined, but remember that cooked flesh is a damaged protein and therefore not an ideal source. Among the flesh products, organic free-range eggs and fish are easiest on the body and therefore better for weight loss and energy. On this note, consider these words from Henry David Thoreau in *Walden*:

> One farmer says to me, "You cannot live on vegetable food solely, for it furnishes nothing to make the bones with"; and so he religiously devotes a part of his day to supplying himself with the raw material of bones; walking all the while he talks behind his oxen, which, with vegetable-made bones, jerk him and his lumbering plow along in spite of every obstacle.

What should I do about my serious sweet tooth?

There are so many delicious sweets included in the program, such as dates, dried fruits, pure maple syrup, Stevia, and agave nectar. You can also enjoy the 70 percent Green & Black chocolate bars, Goldie's carob bars, and Kollar cookies (kollarcookies.com)! Pure maple syrup, Stevia, and agave nectar are all *neutral* sweeteners, so use them to make anything sweeter! When you learn that the ideal food for humans is raw fruit, you start to see why we all have this built-in sweet tooth—so revel in all the sweetness of nature!

If I "fall off the wagon" one day and eat the wrong things in the wrong combinations, is there anything I can do to make up for it?

Absolutely! First of all, if you're going to mess up, you're better off doing so at the last meal of the day rather than early or in the middle of the day. This way you won't incur a pile-up on top of a miscombined meal. If you do eat poorly in the middle of the day, just stick to veggies for dinner. If you're careful not to make two consecutive mistakes one day after the next, you won't backslide. But, even if you fall off for several days, just do the best you can to get back on track again as soon as possible.

I am an avid athlete. Am I going to have enough energy on this program?

Athletes do very well if they approach raw food in the right way. First, focusing on getting the combinations right will give you a lot more energy. As you gradually incorporate more raw foods into your diet, you should have plenty of energy and perform better than ever. Just be sure to eat hearty portions, particularly in the evening.

The raw Lara bars are excellent energy bars for you. You'll find the Kamut pasta and sweet potatoes make excellent substitutes for the white pastas most athletes consume—so enjoy them if you find them helpful, even though they are not raw. If you feel sluggish, it's probably due to a buildup of waste in your bowel. Finding a good colon therapist will make all the difference!

You'll get plenty of protein from your Life Force Power-ade, raw nuts, sea vegetables, and raw goat cheese, and you may also include some organic eggs and fish (preferably for dinner) if you desire. Transition gradually into this program, and you'll have fantastic results. I am extremely active myself and work with many successful athletes who would never go back to protein shakes and power bars! Try the Pumkin Pie in a Bowl (page 166) and the Raw Cream of Tomato Soup (page 167) as pre-workout fuel. These blended soups will give you lots of enzymes without weighing you down. Dates and raw honey-sweetened macaroons are good for fuel stops. And, of course, deep breathing is key!

I'm on a strict budget and concerned about the cost of this diet. Any suggestions?

You don't have to buy the high-end raw food products or the expensive specialty raw treats for this to succeed. It's easy to keep costs down by sticking with green salads, steamed veggies, sweet potatoes, millet, quinoi, sprouted-grain bread, and avocados with some fish when you want it. You can juice tons of organic carrots, which are very cheap. Fresh fruit in season is not expensive. Keep the diet simple, clean, and high in vegetable content.

I lost weight when I first started this diet, but for the past week my scale hasn't budged. What's happening?

The first thing to ask yourself is: "Are my bowels moving on a real regular basis?" If not, that's probably the problem. In addition to taking steps to improve elimination (such as using a stool to prop your feet up, and transitioning more gradually to this predominantly raw food diet), I would limit or eliminate fruit and grains for a week and see what happens. While a clean body will thrive on fruit, fruit can be too cleansing for some people and tie up their bowels. For most women, fish is more slimming than grain, so don't get hung up on the vegetarian ideal, unless you're practicing it for spiritual or ethical reasons.

It's also possible that you're experiencing a brief hiatus as your body readjusts to this new way of eating. It will take some time for your body to cleanse itself of all the excess weight (remember Weight = Waste). As your body experiences deeper healing, the weight will continue to come off!

How do you feed your kids?

My kids eat a huge variety of raw as well as high-quality cooked foods. They love the sprouted-grain bread products, spelt, kamut, and soba noodle pastas as well as sweet potatoes, steamed veggies, and legume-based soups. My son also really enjoys organic eggs. I did keep them totally raw for their first 18 months of life and to this day they have never needed an antibiotic or suffered from ear infections. However, I was able to do this because I was breast-feeding them and knew exactly how to use and incorporate plant foods, greens, and the right sources of plant fats. There are people who attempt to raise vegan or raw babies and fail miserably—not because they are wrong in theory, but because they get it wrong in practice. Please don't use your child as a raw experiment. If you wish to raise your child this way, get a good, knowledgeable health coach who can communicate with you and your doctor.

I believe in allowing for compromises and giving children space to experience tastes and foods that may make us health-conscious adults wince. My method is to be really open with my kids about how the body works and why I choose to eat and feed them this way. I don't forbid them to eat anything, but I do tell them what the effects of certain foods are and why mommy doesn't eat them. I feel good about passing this information on to my children. It is a critical component of their education. And I know that eating this way contributes to their joyful dispositions, which is the best reason in the world to do it!

It helps that many of their friends' parents are following this program and feeding their kids similarly. I see clusters of families creating this kind of community for their children all over the country, which should inspire any parents reading this book!

Are you 100 percent raw?

I do include some steamed veggies and sweet potatoes and the occasional piece of fish when I desire it. I typically take in large amounts of vegetable juice like the Life Force Power-ade (page 158), lots of fresh fruits, and big raw salads. I'm particularly fond of Suddenly St. Tropez (page 179) followed by some dark chocolate. When I'm with friends at a good restaurant, however, I can knock back a couple of glasses of wine and polish off an entrée of fresh fish and veggies following a green salad. I'll even dig into a few bites of ice cream if it's on the dessert menu.

You'll see there's plenty of room to express your eating pleasure and style, even at the highest levels of this diet. A lot of die-hard raw foodists would be critical of this approach, but my goal is clean cells and a body rich with Life Force Energy, not conforming to a label for the sake of being officially "raw." What keeps me going strong year after year is the freedom to always have what I want. I can do this because (1) I flood my body with fresh raw, mostly green vegetable juice every day; (2) I don't take anything into my body until I've ensured that yesterday's waste has passed through me; (3) I always properly combine my meals; and (4) I body brush daily and incorporate colon cleansing as needed every month. I have been living this way for many years and I feel healthier and leaner than I have since I was a kid. In fact, I just keep feeling better and better!

How does this program work for people who suffer from irritable bowel syndrome (IBS)?

Every client I have worked with who has IBS has had great success! The food combining alone should help you tremendously. Once your bowel starts to heal, you will begin eliminating normally. It may take a while, but it will happen. Blended foods are helpful. Fruits may be too cleansing for you at this time and give you trouble. Steamed veggies, vegetable soups, avocados, young coconut, sweet potatoes, and light fish will be easiest on your system right now. Keep your combos straight and you'll see great results!

Can I follow this diet if I have diabetes?

Yes, many diabetics enjoy this program and experience fabulous results! The key is to limit the fruit in the beginning (as you get healthier, you'll be able to eat more fruit) to melons, grapefruit, berries, and green apples, and don't go overboard with the grain items. When you eat sweet potatoes and grains, be sure to have them with hydrating vegetables.

Instead of using maple syrup, you can use small amounts of agave nectar and you can always use Stevia to sweeten a dish without raising blood sugar levels. It's okay to have a few dates here and there in recipes, but don't eat them "straight" in any substantial qualities. There is much to eat other than the very sweet items, so enjoy those other things and focus on great big raw salads with avocados and great dressings (honey is okay in dressing since the abundant water content in the raw vegetables will dilute the sweetness), nut butters, fish, and so on. And always eat in proper combos. The 70-percent chocolate by Green & Black is a perfect dessert for you.

I have a history of *Candida.* How should I tailor this program?

I would steer clear of fruit, sugars, and grains. It would be helpful to go without any sugars, grains, or fermented products for two solid weeks to help wipe out the yeast (at least a large part of it). My clients have had a lot of success doing this while also incorporating the Garden of Life Fungal Defense product and oil of oregano (OregaMax is a good brand). You can take them as recommended while you follow this "*Candida* version" of the diet. Most people do have some fungal growth in their body, so it's probably a good idea for everyone to follow this type of two-week anti-fungal diet once in a while. I do it once a year myself. I would avoid fruit and sugar for two weeks while taking the fungal defense. You will eventually be able to enjoy fruit again once your body is cleaner. Focus on steamed veggies, fish, raw veggies, raw cheese, and sea veggies.

I am terribly addicted to diet soda and could easily drink three liters a day. So while I have little problem eating almost completely raw and in proper quick-exit combinations, I am still very dependent on diet soda. Do you have any suggestions?

The Synergy Grape or Citrus Kombucha can be very helpful when weaning off sodas. You can add more Stevia for sweetness. These beverages are great, bubbly, and will support the healing of your digestive tract! Some of my clients who avoid alcohol enjoy the Kombucha in place of wine.

I love this program but my skin is breaking out. Is there a connection? What can I do?

Your skin is your largest organ and one of the major eliminative organs. If your bowel were cleansed regularly, your skin would be clear almost all the time. You are drawing up more waste than is exiting your system so your body is pushing it out through your skin. Body brushing, saunas, enemas, and/or colonics are the best remedies for this.

I have a very delicate digestive system. I've struggled for years with Crohn's disease and diverticulitis. Can I eat this way?

People with this condition can enjoy lots of Life Force Energy–rich foods if they are well blended. Blended foods are far easier on the digestive tract. In time, your system should regain its strength. Fruit is fine because it's easy to digest, but eat it in moderation because, given your condition, your system is probably too toxic to absorb too much fruit right now. Blend your salads and soups (both raw and cooked), and have virtually no fleshes (occasionally, scrambled eggs or tender, easy-to-digest fish such as sea bass and cod are okay). Avoid all unblended nuts, but you may have small amounts of raw nut-butters.

When I eat a quick-exit meal and feel hungry about an hour later, am I really hungry?

It's likely that what you're experiencing is not hunger, but a literal emptiness. Most people are not used to feeling empty in this way so quickly after a meal. It may take some time to get accustomed to your cleaner, lighter body. When you eat quick-exit meals, you should feel balanced and calm internally. If, however, you are feeling light-headed, that is a cue to eat or drink something that will provide natural sugars to your brain and bloodstream.

How safe is this program for someone who has struggled with an eating disorder?

First, let's establish the fact that there are very few people in our culture who do not have an eating disorder. Some of them are conscious of it and others are not—that is the only difference. The constant consumption of unfit foods is a very real form of disordered eating. Copious consumption of food and television simultaneously is a food and entertainment addiction that is highly disruptive to the human body and spirit. However, I take it you are referring directly to the disorders we call "anorexia," "bulimia," and "obsessive overeating."

I do not agree with the mainstream approach to healing eating disorders—making sure that anorexics and bulimics eat unfit foods—often laden with white flour and corn syrup, just so long as they reach a certain caloric intake and number on the scale. The clinics that attempt to help these people serve the most abominable fare and seem to prioritize weight gain to the exclusion of all other considerations. This approach shows a real ignorance about the larger problem at work, which is usually psychologically and chemically rooted. A few eating disorder clinics are beginning to integrate more holistic practices and cuisine, which is a good sign, but still a far cry from the help these people need.

I have worked with numerous eating-disordered clients, all of whom repeatedly told me that eating this way helped them transform their relationship with food, mainly because their bodies were given a chance to come back into balance. They learned the beautifying, slimming power of truly energizing, life-giving foods, and best of all they shed their negative associations with food and were able to enjoy eating again!

In my opinion, this diet offers the ideal approach for anyone coming from an "eating disorder" mind-set. People often develop eating disorders from a desire to cleanse and strip away the layers of shame and negativity from past lives or deep-rooted emotional issues and chemical reactions to foods. This diet can help heal the body and spirit. However, if you are using this diet as another way for you to act out an extreme form of control over your food intake, it is not going to help you grow any closer to the balance and harmony that the program is about. In that case, I would highly recommend finding at least one good counselor from an appropriate field (whether it's a doctor, psychologist, nutritionist, or a spiritual guide) to help you work through the deeper issues at the root of your disordered eating.

I am a little concerned about the colonics part. I have never done it before and do not feel the need to start now, as I've always been very regular. Is it really necessary?

Colonics are just one of those things that are necessary for reaching the highest levels of health and energy, even for those who consider themselves to be "regular." I believe colonics will be considered as essential to the maintenance of the body as brushing your teeth in a decade's time. It's one of those things you will only understand once you undergo a series of colonics in conjunction with this diet program. A gravity enema is good as well if you cannot get a colonic right away.

Can I use my high-powered blender instead of the juicer to make vegetable juice? Is it really better than an ordinary mixer? I really don't want to spend the money on a juicer.

A juicer is completely different from a blender. In my opinion, both are necessary kitchen appliances, but for very different tasks. A juicer separates the fiber from the precious organic liquid of the plant. So, in order to benefit from the true power of the vegetable elixirs, you must use a juicer. Meanwhile, blenders are essential for making dressings, soups, and ice creams, which you cannot make with a juicer. Juicers don't have to be terribly expensive. In fact, my favorite juicer is the Breville brand. They have several models, which are all good, retailing for as low as $100 and as much as $350. You can find them online at www.therawfooddetoxdiet.com.

I would like to add more raw food in my diet but do not want to lose weight. In fact, is there any way to gain weight on this program?

If you want to attain a healthy weight, your tissue quality needs to improve. This means that for a time as you detox you may lose weight. Imagine a sponge being squeezed and made very small, but then expanding back to its true size once the junk is squeezed out of it. Try to focus less on your weight and more on your journey to cellular health! In the meantime, you won't have to worry so much about food combinations or consuming too many raw fats or cooked grains. Enjoy all of the natural foods liberally! If your natural, healthy weight is higher than it is now, you will get there eventually—but it may take some time.

I noticed that you incorporate a lot of high-glycemic-index foods such as bananas, maple syrup, dates, and 70 percent chocolate bars. How is it possible to eat a large quantity of these types of foods without spiking your blood sugar level up and causing weight gain?

It's always hard for people to accept that some of the foods they have previously learned to shun for health and weight reasons happen to be the healthiest and best options for energy and weight loss. As I've said before, unless you have a medical condition that limits your intake of fresh and dried fruits, raw honey, and so on, you can feel great about eating all of these foods, despite where they may fall on the glycemic index. The glycemic index is helpful but it does not tell the whole story.

The 70 percent chocolate bars, nuts, cold-pressed oils, avocados, and coconuts are high in fat. Shouldn't these sorts of foods be consumed in moderation?

The answer really depends on your gender. Ladies, I'm sorry, but we don't break down fats very well (men don't really have to measure their raw fat intake too much until they become much, much cleaner). However, we can still eat fairly abundant amounts of raw fats like the ones mentioned above. For example, you can eat a whole avocado and pour on the dressings in this book, enjoy half a dark chocolate bar, and a good portion of your favorite nut-based raw treats. You can eat these particular raw fats with no ill effects because they are easily recognized, digested, and eliminated by the body. As long as you don't gorge on them, they will not leave behind waste. Cooked fats, on the other hand, are not recognized by the body and sit in the cells, weighing you down, causing illness, and zapping your energy!

I've always heard it is better to eat dinner early, but my schedule and lifestyle have me eating around 9 or 10 P.M. Will this interfere with my progress?

You'll be happy to know that you do not have to eat an early dinner for this diet to work. As long as you properly combine and eat high–Life Force Energy foods, you may eat as late as you need to. There are two important factors to remember, though: (1) Do not go to sleep on a full stomach; be sure to keep yourself vertical for at least an hour after eating your late dinner meal. (2) Make sure you get adequate sleep. If you're eating dinner at 11 and going to bed after midnight, I hope you're able to sleep past 8 the next morning. You cannot cheat yourself on sleep and expect to give your body the time it needs to heal deeply and recharge.

Of course, many raw foodists brag about needing very little sleep. And indeed, on this diet you may be go through phases of feeling completely rested after only a few hours of sleep, but this is not usually a consistent pattern. An average of eight hours of sleep each night is still a good rule of thumb, especially given the extremely busy lifestyles many of us lead today. Adequate amounts of sleep will help to raise your vibrations and make you more productive and energized during the day. (I have also noticed that my clients tend to stall their weight loss and even backslide when they go for periods of inadequate sleep.) So, eat late and be merry 'til the wee hours—but only if you can back it up with a full sleep cycle.

There are many colon-cleansing kits and herbal formulas for bowel cleansing. Should I be using them?

I do not recommend using herbal laxatives. While they will stimulate bowel evacuations for beginners, they achieve this by irritating the intestines and releasing only the superficial matter—never reaching the deep impacted matter. Almost any cleansing method will work for a beginner because the body isn't used to bowel stimulation, but they will eventually stop working. By this point, people are either addicted to them—needing more and more of it to work, which causes much intestinal strife, or give up and return to their previous food-lifestyle. The reason these products sell so well is because people love to see things work—even if only initially. It gives them hope.

If you want to use an herbal laxative in the beginning, just for the initial stage, and then move on to colonics, that is an option. But runny, watery stools are an indication of deep constipation and a highly irritated intestine, not of efficient waste removal. Colonics are a whole different ball game. They simply hydrate the colon with pure water and, getting into deep recesses of the colon walls, carry out the old, impacted waste matter, leaving you feeling lighter and cleaner with each treatment. Many find that aloe vera products can help soften and prepare the waste matter for evacuation by colonics and natural means.

You spoke about the link between vibrations and energy in the first part of this book. I've heard it said that every color has a different vibration. How do colors and eating the "rainbow" of colors in nature fit into this approach?

Every color has a specific vibration. If we look at the seven basic colors of the visible light spectrum (the rainbow), we see that there is a progression in the vibratory rate, starting with red, the slowest (oscillating with a wavelength of about 650 to 700 nanometers in length) to violet, the fastest (oscillating with a wavelength of about 400 nanometers). The chakra system (as explained on page 75) is also intimately linked with color and the vibrational sway of each color; not only does each chakra correspond to a particular color, but the color progression of the chakra system is identical to that of the visible light spectrum. The seven energy centers in the chakra system and their corresponding colors are as follows: chakra 1, the base (or root) chakra, which lies at the base of the spine, is red; chakra 2, the sacral chakra, which lies just below the belly button, is orange; chakra 3, the solar plexus chakra located about two inches above the navel, is yellow; chakra 4, the heart chakra, located in the center of the chest, is green; chakra 5, the throat chakra, located in the center of the throat, is blue; chakra 6, the third-eye chakra, located between the eyes, is indigo; and chakra 7, the crown chakra, located at the crown of the head, is violet. This shows us that from our base to our crown, our energy body is like a rainbow. If we are in balance and our energy is flowing well, we are nothing less radiant than a walking, talking rainbow of light energy!

Since the goal is to feed the energy body, which is made up of vibrationally active color, we need to feed our bodies a rainbow of colorful foods every day to ensure that each part of our energy body (each chakra center) is fully nourished.

Many raw food enthusiasts seem to overdose on raw fats. A raw foodist could easily devote a large percentage of their diet to fat (oils, nuts, seeds, avocados, etc.). How much fat is optimal on a raw or high-raw diet, and how much is too much?

Men and women digest fats differently. Whereas most men will not have any problem with normal amounts of raw fats, women do not break them down nearly as well. Women must be very careful about overeating nuts, coconut butter, and raw oils. I have noticed among my female colleagues and clients that those women who take in very little fat and are careful not to mix fats (such as olive oil with avocado, or nuts with oils) do the best in the long term.

Aspiring raw foodists wind up eating too much fat due to a lack of proper transition, which makes them desperate for the dense stimulation that their old diet provided. These people are simply trying to replicate their old favorite foods in raw-food form. For example, they replace cheeseburgers with nut burgers or potato chips with pounds of raw nuts. This strong desire for dense, fatty foods is curtailed when one uses transition foods like sprouted-grain bread products, baked sweet potatoes with organic butter, fish, and cooked vegetables. I would sooner eat three baked sweet potatoes with a green salad in one sitting than a pound of raw macadamias. I would sooner eat a filet of striped bass than a smoothie filled with raw coconut butter (coconut butter is much denser and harder on the liver than many cooked-food choices). A person who transitions properly away from the standard American diet (SAD) will not overdose on raw fats because they will be gently weaning themselves of their old chemical and psychological addictions.

Do people need to make a special effort to get the essential fats—for example, by taking flax oil or ground flaxseeds for omega-3 fatty acids? Or can adequate amounts of all of the essential fats be obtained just through eating a varied raw diet, without the need for concentrated sources? Do you, personally, make a point of eating specific foods on a daily basis in order to obtain specific essential fats?

Contrary to all the hype around flax and fish oils, there is no benefit to taking in extra oils, flaxseeds, and so on. They are difficult to break down, and the average aspiring raw foodist is going to get more than enough "good fat" from a day's worth of raw meals. Use raw oils for creating delicious salads. Let's not turn them into some kind of miracle food and encourage the consumption of more dense fats that will only slow you and your cleansing process down.

I notice you recommend eating bananas, but I understand that they are binding. Isn't there a contradiction here?

Unripe bananas are binding. However, fully ripe bananas (with no green on the ends) actually have a laxative effect. The problem is that people often eat bananas before they are ripe, which is why bananas have this unfortunate reputation.

Was it always easy for you to eat this way?

It may help you to know that I did not always eat this way or even think I ever could. I can even remember when, more than ten years ago, one of my friends was undertaking a week-long detox, eating only fruits and vegetables. I was in awe of her self-discipline, of her ability to go a whole week without eating cheese, flesh foods, frozen yogurt, or bread. Many of these foods were staples of my diet back then. To keep my weight in check, I used to think I had to eat grilled chicken every day for lunch and some variation of it or other flesh protein for dinner, which wound up making me feel very dependent on those foods for a feeling of fullness at mealtime. I had already struggled with my weight and body image throughout my teenage years and found the prospect of struggling with them for the rest of my life exhausting and downright depressing. Between the self-loathing, the hours I spent at the gym, and the effort and expense I put into creating a wardrobe to mask my "wobbly bits," it was a full-time preoccupation!

I understand that there is a lot of information here that may sound too restrictive because I felt the same way back then. I was not born with a special gene that made it easier for me to adopt this diet lifestyle than anyone else. I had just as many food addictions and bad habits as the next person. The trick was to take it all in at my own pace. I just gradually dipped into this "pool of energy" until one day I looked around and realized I could swim—and it was really fun and fulfilling to boot!

HIERARCHY OF VIBRATIONAL NUTRITION

Below are the frequency ranges of basic foods as measured by the Tainio Technology Frequency Monitoring Device (currently the most accurate tool for measuring food frequencies). Remember, this device *does not* distinguish between harmonious and inharmonious vibrations. This is why animal fleshes can register higher than sprouted grains and cooked vegetables. The Hierarchy of Foods chart on page 22 takes everything into account—harmony, ease of digestion, alkalinity, and vibrational values. Use that chart to determine the health, energy, and weight loss values of the foods you eat. I'm providing this chart just to give you the scientific vibrational measurements of common foods. For the purposes of this chart, "raw" refers to plant foods that have not been heated above 118° F.

Fresh fruits (organic and picked when ripe) ....80 MHz

Raw green vegetables (organic)..65–72 MHz

Fish (wild)..50–55 MHz

Fish (farmed) ....40–45 MHz

Wine ....40–50 MHz

Chicken (organic, free range)...40–45 MHz

Beef (organic, grass fed) ....40–45 MHz

Sprouted grains ....35–45 MHz

Chicken (caged) ....20–25 MHz

Pork...15–20 MHz

Beef (mainstream)..15–20 MHz

Raw nongreen vegetables, including root vegetables (organic) ....13–21 MHz

Processed sprouted-grain products (sprouted-grain breads) ....10–15 MHz

Cooked vegetables (inorganic boiled vegetables
are at the lower end of the vibration spectrum;
organic steamed vegetables are at the higher end) ....7–25 MHz

Cheeseburger..5–10 MHz

Nuts (raw) ....5–7 MHz

Nuts (roasted, processed)...1–2 MHz

Grains (refined, such as white
flour and refined grain products)...< 1 MHz
(in the low kilohertz range)

Fast food french fries ....< 1 MHz
(in the low kilohertz range)

RECOMMENDED READING

Aihara, Herman. *Acid & Alkaline*. Chico, CA: George Ohsawa Macrobiotic Foundation, 1986.

Baroody, Theodore A. *Alkalinize or Die*. Waynesville, NC: Holographic Health Press, 1991.

Clark, Glenn. *The Man Who Tapped the Secrets of the Universe*. Waynesboro, VA: The University of Science and Philosophy, 1946.

Cousense, Gabriel. *Spiritual Nutrition: Six Foundations for Spiritual Life and the Awakening of Kundalini*, Berkeley, CA: North Atlantic Books, 2005.

Dyer, Wayne W. *Inspiration: Your Ultimate Calling*. Carlsbad, CA: Hay House Publishing, 2006.

Ehret, Arnold. *The Mucusless Diet & Healing System*. New York, NY: Benedict Lust Publications, 1922.

Gerber, Richard. *Vibrational Medicine*. Rochester, VT: Bear & Company, 2001.

Hills, Christopher. *Nuclear Evolution: Discovery of the Rainbow Body*, Boulder Creek, CO: University of the Trees Press, 1977.

Hunt, Valerie V. *Infinite Mind: Science of the Human Vibrations of Consciousness*. Malibu, CA: Malibu Publishing Company, 1989.

Kit, Wong Kiew. *The Art of Chi Kung*. New York, NY: Cosmos Publishing, 1993.

Kulvinskas, Viktoras. *Survival into the 21st Century*. Woodstock Valley, CT: Omangod Press, 1975.

Murphy, Michael. *The Future of the Body: Explorations into the Further Evolution of Human Nature*, New York, NY: Putnam, 1993.

Russell, Walter. *A New Concept of the Universe*. Waynesboro, VA: The Walter Russell Foundation, The University of Science and Philosophy, 1989.

Walker, Norman. *Raw Vegetable Juices: What's Missing in Your Body*. Prescott, AZ: Norwalk Press, 1977.

Walker, Norman. *Colon Health: The Key to a Vibrant Life*. Prescott, AZ: Norwalk Press, 1979.

Wilber, Ken. *The Spectrum of Consciousness*. Wheaton, IL: Quest Books, 1977.

INDEX

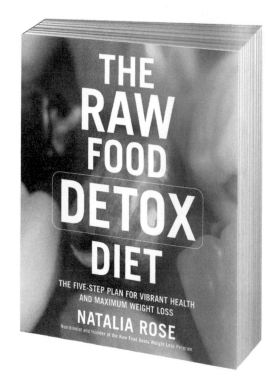
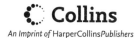